Praise for *Normal Broken*

"*Normal Broken* is the rare book about grief that tells the whole truth without empty platitudes and welcomes readers at any stage of grieving. Kelly Cervantes's loving and often hilarious voice guides readers by drawing on her own experience of loss and offering the wisdom she learned while traveling through grief's dark tunnel. The real gift of this book is that it offers hope and company for losses of all sizes and shapes, and I know I will return to it for years to come."

—Christie Tate, author of *New York Times* bestselling *GROUP* and *BFF*

"Kelly Cervantes gently leads us through our own unique grief journey with compassion, empathy, and heart. Feeling broken together is what binds us in this human experience, and *Normal Broken* shows us beautifully how to do that for each other and ourselves."

—Meredith Ethington, author of *The Mother Load*

"More than a poignant memoir, *Normal Broken* is a validating friend for anyone laden with grief. Whether we are in the acute, early days of loss or dreading yet another chronic milestone, this book offers support and solidarity without judgment or agenda. Informed by her hard-earned insights, Kelly Cervantes beautifully unburdens grievers with permissions we didn't know we needed and subtly models a mini but mighty micro-measurement to help us inch toward healing."

—Stephanie Sarazin, author of *Soulbroken*

"Stunning. Heartbreaking. Beautiful. Thank you, Kelly, for helping us heal."

—Leslie Means, founder and owner of Her View From Home and author of *Wall Street Journal* bestselling *God Made a Mother*

"In *Normal Broken*, Kelly Cervantes chronicles a mother's heart-wrenching journey of having, loving, and ultimately losing her firstborn daughter, Adelaide. While I've certainly experienced loss, I've never known the magnitude of grief that comes from experiencing child loss. My only concern going into this book was that I might struggle to relate, but ten minutes later, I'd opened a highlighter and yelled for the kids to pipe down. *Normal Broken* is so much more than a mother's journey toward healing. It's a survivor's guide for the scariest, twistiest valley of the human experience—loss. Unafraid of her own grief (or a delightfully dark joke), Cervantes writes with the Band-Aid off and shows us the process of healing. Part breathtaking, part heartbreaking, and 100-percent full of hope, *Normal Broken* is here for the grief conversation with the much-needed voice of a friend."

—Mary Katherine Backstrom, author of *Crazy Joy* and *Holy Hot Mess*

"Harrowingly transparent, Kelly Cervantes's soul-baring *Normal Broken* is a dear companion for those who are suffering, a glimmer of hope when all seems lost, and a poignantly delivered reminder that even when mired in the chaos of grief, we are not alone. It is essential reading for those who are struggling to endure the unimaginable."

—Daniel Lerner, coauthor of *U Thrive*

Normal Broken

THE GRIEF COMPANION
FOR WHEN IT'S TIME
TO HEAL BUT YOU'RE NOT
SURE YOU WANT TO

KELLY CERVANTES

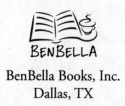

BenBella Books, Inc.
Dallas, TX

BenBella Books, Inc.
10440 N. Central Expressway
Suite 800
Dallas, TX 75231
benbellabooks.com
Send feedback to feedback@benbellabooks.com

BenBella is a federally registered trademark.

Printed in the United States of America
10 9 8 7 6 5 4 3 2 1

Library of Congress Control Number: 2023013938
ISBN 9781637743829 (trade paperback)
ISBN 9781637743836 (electronic)

Editing by Alyn Wallace
Copyediting by Leah Baxter
Proofreading by Lisa Story and Ashley Casteel
Text design and composition by PerfecType, Nashville, TN
Cover design by Sarah Avinger
Cover images © by Ira E (leaf) and Vincent van Zalinge (ladybug) on Unsplash
Printed by Lake Book Manufacturing

Special discounts for bulk sales are available. Please contact bulkorders@benbellabooks.com.

For the broken.
In memory of Adelaide and all the bugs.

Contents

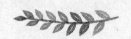

Introduction

> Life is pain, Highness. Anyone who says differently is
> selling something.
>
> —William Goldman

Grief sucks. It's also weird. Basically, it sucks and it's weird. It also happens to be an unavoidable part of life.

Did you know that there is a Grief Awareness Day? It's August 30th, if you were curious. I remember discovering that and wondering who were the lucky prats that were so untouched by grief that they needed to have a day in order to be aware of it. If you are reading these opening lines, I can only assume that you do not fall into that category. I'm so sorry you're not one of the lucky prats, but I am glad you're here.

I came to write this book a bit begrudgingly. Not because I didn't believe that it needed to be written, but because I knew how difficult it would be to write: let's sit in all my worst emotions and memories, and analyze how they affected me and what I learned from them. Sounds like an anxiety attack waiting to happen, right? Thankfully, I've kept a blog since 2018 chronicling much of the major grief I've experienced, so I was able to reexamine the state of mind I had at the time. What I discovered surprised me.

In so many ways I still feel beleaguered and broken by my losses, but time's persistent trudge forward has dragged me along, too. Returning to my blogs allowed me to see how far I've come. My once-fresh wounds have scabbed over, my endurance in daily life has strengthened, and I am no longer living life from moment to moment. Sure, sometimes I find myself picking at those scabs, gushing grief all over again, or I push myself too far and land back in a fetal position, tapped of physical and emotional energy. But I am *healing*.

That was a significant discovery, considering that early in my grief journey I wasn't sure that I wanted to heal. My daughter Adelaide passed away in 2019, five days shy of her fourth birthday, but I had been grieving her long before she left us. In May 2016, the same week my husband landed the lead role of Hamilton in the brand-new Chicago production of the blockbuster musical, our daughter was diagnosed with epilepsy. She was only seven months old at the time and would be wracked by seizures for the rest of her brief life. They were years that my husband, Miguel, would compare to holding on to a rocket in one hand while dragging a parachute behind you with the other.

Several months before she passed, doctors determined that whatever was causing Adelaide's seizures was neurodegenerative and there was nothing else that could be done to help her. By the time she died, I felt like a professional griever. It was a routine part of my day. I had grieved the milestones she missed, the words she never spoke, the smiles she forfeited, and the entire life I had dreamed for her—all before I ever grieved her physical loss. Not that any of this made her death any easier to process, though, admittedly, I had hoped it might (more on that later).

Then, only days after Adelaide died, my grief was compounded when we learned Miguel would take over as Hamilton on Broadway. This meant leaving our beloved Chicago community to return to New York City after three years away. What should have been amazing news (being Hamilton in *Hamilton* on Broadway!!!), I would instead view as taking us away from our supportive friends, who had known Adelaide better than anyone else. Five months later, in March 2020, just ten performances into Miguel's Broadway run, the world was thrown into collective quarantine. At this point, I was fairly confident that I had been cast in some sort of cosmic shit show.

Not only did my grief become destructive, but I had absolutely zero interest in healing, perhaps because for much of Adelaide's life my love for her got tangled up in the emotional pain I experienced at the hands of her medical condition. If I tried to heal, that would require me to let go of the pain and, by extension, I thought, my daughter. I hadn't been able to physically keep Adelaide in our lives, so you better believe I had no intention of letting go of her emotionally, ergo the attachment to pain.

Yet everywhere I turned, I felt like healing thoughts, vibes, and prayers were being flung in my direction. It took time, intense reflection, and a heavy dose of anti-depressants for me to understand that healing was going to happen whether I wanted it to or not. Time heals, it just does. Ready or not, here it comes, and in its wake we are left with scars. Scars we are taught to hide away—which is probably why I equated healing with forgetting.

But our scars aren't something to be embarrassed by or insecure about. They are reminders of battles fought—so why not accept and own the lines of the scar? What if instead of burying the scars under clothes and fake smiles, we displayed them with honor and remembrance? What if you could turn your jagged, tough skin into a work of art by designing a beautiful tattoo around it? That, to me, is healing: the reminders of the pain are still there, but the marks they leave behind and the person we become as a result pay homage to a life lived. After all, the only reason loss hurts so much is because we love so hard. There is no loss without love, and there is nothing more beautiful (or complicated) in this world than love. So, it stands to reason that we should be able to find beauty, and even create beauty, out of our losses.

Through writing and sharing my blog, *Inchstones*, I discovered—even during some of my darkest moments—that I was far from alone in my thoughts and experiences. I also discovered that I'm pretty good at putting those often-irrational feelings into words so that others could relate to and identify with them. I didn't start writing the blog to help others. It was part of my own therapeutic journey, a way to process my life in eight-hundred-word weekly installments. But it did help others, and knowing that, in turn, helped me feel that maybe all this pain didn't need to be in vain. *Normal Broken* was born out of this desire to lend a hand and help others find their own words.

Even if that means simply sitting in the dark together, acknowledging our brokenness, and feeling broken together.

What you can expect from this book are honest pieces of my personal story and the candid realizations I made along the way that helped me survive and, yes, even heal. You probably won't connect with everything here because we all grieve differently—and that's okay! I would never presume to tell anyone how to grieve, but I do hope that you can pull nuggets from my trials and insights that can help make your own grief journey a little less treacherous. Or, at the very least, feel you are not navigating it alone.

Another thing you should know about this book is that, while it is segmented into chapters because that is how books work, that does not mean that I've discovered some magical order to healing. Grief is many things, but linear is not one of them. Just as what we are grieving varies, so does how we process it. Please feel free to take these chapters in whatever order you need as you navigate your grief. Let this book meet you where you are at whatever moment you happen to arrive there.

While I'm dismantling how books are read, let me also confess that self-help books have never been my jam. I've never dealt well with people telling me what to do—even as a child I insisted on learning by doing everything myself ("I do it! I do it!"). So, in this book you will not find boldfaced type with bullet-pointed advice, because I could never write a book that I wouldn't read myself. I should also add that I am not a therapist, counselor, or social worker, and this book is not to be confused with psychiatric guidance. I am a typical woman who has experienced unimaginable loss and is *still* stumbling through my grief. Which, I hope, makes this book accessible and approachable. So, expect more of *this helped me* and less of *research shows this is what healthy grieving should look like.* These pages are not meant to be a guide. Instead, think of them as a companion to support you during a super-shitty time in your life.

However, I do have one kind of self-help-adjacent trick that I suggest trying: writing. By putting words to my most hollowing emotions and confusing thoughts, I have been able to blow away the oppressive grief fog more effectively than a high-powered fan in a Beyoncé music video. Look, I'm not going to tell you to drink less and exercise more because, well, duh. I'm also not about to bore you with statistics about how journaling benefits mood, memory, sleep, and self-confidence.[1] But this writing thing? I'm pretty passionate about it.

There is so much power in putting our trials and triumphs into words—in naming what drives our conscious thoughts. Aside from a few dependable humans and one devoted canine, writing is the thing that is most responsible for my progress. But because I am well aware of how daunting a blank page can be, I have included writing prompts after each chapter where you can add your own thoughts, lists, or revelations. The prompts include questions and ideas that have swirled in my head over time and will hopefully jumpstart different trains of thought and streams of consciousness in you as you continue on your own journey. If this makes you cringe or roll your eyes, I feel you. But I really do recommend giving it a try, and if you hate it, no worries. Just pretend like those pages don't even exist in the book and move on to the next. You're not going to hurt my feelings. You do you.

Oh! One last thing I need you to know: grief should never be a competition. Mark Twain said, "Nothing that grieves us can be called little: by the eternal laws of proportion a child's loss of a doll and a king's loss of a crown are events of the same size."[2] Whether you are showing up today having lost a parent, spouse, friend, or child; whether you are grieving your previous life, a career, a version of yourself, or a future life you had envisioned; whether you are grieving someone who is deeply alive but so very far away—your grief is valid. If you find this concept challenging because you believe that your loss pales in comparison to others', or, conversely, you are growing ever more annoyed with those who you perceive as suffering from less than you are, I recommend flipping ahead to Chapter 11: When Gratitude Is a Struggle, where we take on comparative and competitive grief. Our feelings are justified by our lived experiences and resulting perspective: one person's toy is another person's kingdom, and that principle must be honored without judging others or, perhaps more commonly, judging ourselves. We cannot expect to heal if we are concerned about how our grief fits into a fictitious hierarchy of our own design.

Alright then. With all that out of the way, let's try to start suturing our wounds and creating works of art out of these hard-earned scars.

1

When Getting Out of Bed
Deserves a Medal

I told her once I wasn't good at anything. She told me
survival is a talent.

—Susanna Kaysen

No one told me how much time I would spend in bed the weeks, months, and years following Adelaide's death. No one told me—or maybe I just wasn't paying attention when they did—how exhausting grief is.

Yes, of course it's emotionally exhausting, but it is also physically and mentally debilitating. Every cell of my body yearned to be horizontal and covered in cotton. It was an exacting feat to rise in the morning, and it required an equally strenuous effort to resist my bed's siren song to return. I often fell victim to its haunting melody, filled with false promises of returning to the days when my daughter was alive. The days when I would lie beside her in her twin bed, snuggle into her neck, and savor the scent of her baby-soft skin. Back when I wondered if all this time I'd already spent grieving her would count as time served. I wasn't a prisoner per se, but I had spent the better part of three years willingly chained to my medically complex daughter. I had grieved the first words never uttered, the first steps never taken, the first day of preschool never attended. There had been plenty of celebrations as well, but the grief was always there, tingeing our best moments together like a bad photo filter. Certainly, all those tears must count for something?

When I told my mental-health-therapist mother about my hope for time-served grief, she smiled gently and all too knowingly before telling me she didn't think it worked that way. That I ought to expect a year or two of intense grief before I began to feel like some semblance of myself again.

A year?! Or *two*?!

What she didn't tell me then, but would clue me in to a few months later, when the concept wasn't quite so overwhelming, was that I would never truly feel like me again. I had been forever changed. I needed to constantly remind myself of that in those first few years. I wasn't pushing forward to get back to who I was, but instead pushing forward to grow into the next version of myself.

Still, after Adelaide passed, and I connected with people who had lost a loved one suddenly as well as those who had known the end was coming, I concluded that my idea of time served *could* apply to those early days after her passing. My years of pre-grieving, if you will, allowed me to hit fast-forward on the shock and acceptance of our lost future in a way those stunned by loss could not and cannot.

Regardless, I am still left with a gaping void where my child used to be. I am still left with an unknown future because my entire existence revolved around her. I am still left with the guilt of acknowledging how much easier our life is now without her physical presence.

I am still left.

My "time served" didn't lessen the pain or the length of my sentence. I just processed it all a little differently than those shocked by their loss. Not better, not worse, just different. We've all been left. The world moves on, creeping forward one excruciating day at a time with no concern for who's taking part.

Making our way through grief can feel like we are swimming through syrup. It is thick, sticky, and gets on everything. Every action takes so much more additional effort. Then, when you look behind you, exhausted and fighting to stay above the surface, you realize you've barely moved from where you were.

And there are the times when no forward motion seems possible. You are stagnant, treading tar. The first time I felt this was a few months after Adelaide had passed. The meal train had concluded, the flowers had long since died and been thrown away, and, aside from the looks of pity in some people's eyes when they greeted me, most everyone else had moved on. I was going to meetings, running errands, and generally doing life, but I felt directionless, purposeless.

When a friend, who had lost her father not too long before we said goodbye to Adelaide, asked where I was in the grieving process, I explained that I had moved past the debilitating phase where slothing is a legitimate activity, but I still felt off. Truer still was that I felt like my own skin was vacant. As if, out in the world, I was wearing a mask of my own face and wondering if anyone could tell. I felt empty. Like I'd taken up residence in some sort of grief limbo: going through the essential motions of life, committing to what was absolutely needed of me, but making no effort to go further. I mean, how did anyone actually expect me to function in this new normal without my daughter?

Then, a few months after speaking with my grieving friend, and after moving eight hundred miles away from all our friends who knew Adelaide best—in the middle of a pandemic—with the one-year anniversary of her death looming in front of me like an F5 tornado ready to destroy all my hard-fought healing, I found myself not just stuck, but actually regressing. I was lost and depressed. I felt broken. Not in a way that could be fixed with a spot of superglue, but irreparably shattered. I had reverted back to slothing.

With most activities and events still on hold and no dire purpose for me within our home, I found little reason to vacate the covers. There was more than one instance where I decided it would be easier if I wasn't alive anymore. I didn't wish for death exactly; I never made plans to carry it out. But my grief was heavier than the air in a crowded sauna, and if there had been a tragic accident that took my life, I would have gone in peace. I decided that Miguel and our then seven-year-old son, Jackson, would be okay without me, eventually.

They already had each other to depend on, which was more than I could guarantee either of them had from me.

Rationally, I knew this feeling was probably normal, though a smidge alarming. I understood that it was important to give myself time to recalibrate; I *got* that this was all part of the process. But at the same time, I was also anxious to get on with it. It wasn't super comfortable existing this way, so how long was this phase going to last? It had been months since my friend had asked me where I was in the grief process—when would I get to feel like me again? Or some new version of me? Was *this* the new version of me? Good lord, I hoped not!

These were all rhetorical questions, of course. No one could give me an answer, especially since the grieving process is different for everyone. But I wanted a finish line and a goal to meet. That was how I had functioned up to this point in my life, whether with sales quotas at my events job or executing treatment plans as Adelaide's caregiver. Where was my checklist, and who was erasing the progress I had made? My life flipped upside down in a single second when Adelaide died. It only seemed fair that it would flip right side up again just as suddenly, no?

What's that you say? Life's not fair? Clearly.

Fair or not, life does tend to give us signs when we are heading in the right direction. Like mile markers or landmarks by which we can navigate. I was driving down the street in our new hometown when I saw a mural on the side of a building that said "SURVIVE." Nothing else, just "SURVIVE" in bright, spray-painted graffiti letters. I clung to that word because grief is something we live with, not so unlike the way someone grappling with addiction lives with their disease. They will say that they're in recovery, but rarely that they have recovered. Similarly, I will never consider myself as a "survivor" or having survived my loss. No, it is a constant effort to survive. Some days the effort is minimal; other days that tornado is barreling straight toward me. But even then, or perhaps especially then, I have to look past the wind-tossed cow flying in front of my windshield and focus on surviving.

But how do you maneuver around that cow and start making forward progress again, especially if your inner compass isn't entirely sure which way forward even is? What I discovered is fairly simple compared to the complexities of grief: choose what feels right now. Don't worry about the future, try not to dwell entirely on the past, and focus on the present and what needs to be done, or what you want to do, in this exact moment.

This means giving yourself permission to be productive when the mood strikes. Have the energy to start that home project that's been on the list for months? Do it! Inspired to clean the bathroom? By all means. Up for a call with a friend? Reach out! My salve was organizing. I love when everything has a place, regardless of whether my children or husband are capable of acknowledging said thing's place. There were dozens of other more pressing tasks on my list, but instead I switched out the seasonal clothes in my closet, cleaned out the junk drawer, and went through the bible-high stack of papers on the desk. Whatever it is that you feel like you can do, do it, and do it free from any corresponding guilt. Don't worry about something else you should be doing. Don't worry about if you're grieving enough or too little or how others might perceive your activity. The important thing is to *do* when doing feels right.

But this also means relieving yourself of similar guilt when you need to crawl back into bed thirty minutes later. It means saying yes to a dinner invitation, but then when the day arrives and the thought of leaving your home has you reaching for your anti-anxiety meds, allowing yourself to cancel.

So lean into those moments of productivity. Because being productive feels good—it gets those endorphins flowing. A ball in motion stays in motion, and all that. But keep in mind that grief doesn't always adhere to the laws of physics, and our balls can roll along quite merrily until they just stop—no signs, no warning, just no more motion. When that happens, give yourself a moment . . . or a nap. Give in to grief's weirder manifestations. For me, that means listening to an audio recording of my daughter's oxygen concentrator. Here is a machine that I'd loathed: big, bulky, noisy, and tethered to Adelaide for the better part of the last year of her life. Then, after she passed, I found no sound more comforting than its bubbling water, puffing air, buzzing motor, and rattling plastic where the casing was coming apart. Like a white noise machine, I fell asleep to it for weeks.

"What helps you sleep? Melatonin? Chamomile tea? A nice warm bath?" someone might have asked. Nope. The sweet, sweet, sounds of a worse-for-wear oxygen concentrator. I imagine it's like someone else listening to mundane old voicemails about picking up more eggs.

Grief is weird. So very, very weird.

I remember people telling me to take it "a day at a time." They clearly did not know how long a day actually was. By choosing whatever feels right *now*, you only need to take the first scootch forward. It's a lesson I had learned early in my daughter's care: focus on inchstones, not milestones. Especially in the early childhood years, people focus so much on your child meeting milestones. But when your child is disabled, those milestones may take longer to achieve or look very different from what you had expected. So, instead of focusing on the milestones of, say, walking, you focus on the inchstones it takes to get there: better head control, or lifting and lowering a foot while in a gait trainer.

For the first two years of Adelaide's life, we lived inchstone to inchstone, noting each time she sat unassisted a few seconds longer than she had the week before or vocalized a new sound or reached more consistently for an object. My concerns were still there, but as long as we were making progress, albeit mind-numbingly slow progress, I stayed hopeful. However, when Adelaide began regressing and our worst nightmare—that her condition was neurode-generative—was confirmed, my original conception of inchstones became cold comfort. It was then that inchstones took on a new meaning for me. Just because I could no longer see even a half-inchstone's worth of progress in Adelaide's development didn't mean that I couldn't *personally* live inchstone to inchstone.

This philosophy carried me through Adelaide's last months and continues to guide me well after her passing. After all, milestones don't stop in childhood; there are graduations and marriages, careers and families. Adelaide taught me how to celebrate my personal inchstones on the way to life's milestones—and this same logic can apply to grief. Celebrate getting out of bed, getting dressed, doing laundry, or leaving the house. Celebrate meeting up with a friend, feeling emotionally stable, or making it through a day without a nap. By focusing on my inchstones, I was able to lighten the weight of life's grander pressures.

It helped me to make a to-do list with the most basic of activities. Celebrating the act of crossing off "brush teeth" may seem like a low bar, but remember those weeks when you couldn't remember the last time you *had* in fact brushed your teeth? This is progress! These are your inchstones! By breaking things down and acknowledging even the smallest bit of progress, we can get an endorphin boost to keep our little ball rolling along.

Allow yourself to celebrate surviving another day, whether that's with a piece of dark chocolate you have stashed away from prying eyes or by listening to their favorite song for the thousandth time. Small goals will inevitably build upon each other, and rewarding yourself is an encouragement to keep going. The tar will loosen around your ankles, and you can move forward again.

While we're giving our minds gold star stickers for everyday tasks, it's also important not to neglect our bodies. In the intro, I promised I wasn't going to tell you to work out more, and I swear that is not where this is headed. It's just that it turns out that grief can take a physical toll on our bodies as well. I'm talking beyond the exhaustion and the weight gain or loss—there can be actual physical ramifications of grief. Dr. Marilyn Mendoza, a clinical instructor at Tulane University and private practice psychologist, found that grief can in fact affect *all twelve* of the body's systems. (For those of you who also fared poorly in your high school human physiology class, those are the cardiovascular, digestive, endocrine, integumentary, immune, lymphatic, muscular, nervous, renal, reproductive, respiratory, and skeletal systems.) Yeah, you read that right. Grief is not just emotional, it can impact every part of our bodies.

"In fact," Dr. Mendoza writes, "during the first four to six months after the loss of a loved one, people are more likely to experience some type of physical problem, with men being at greater risk than women."[3] Essentially, grief is something that we must physically survive. And while grief can pop up anywhere in our bodies, it most commonly affects our immune, digestive, cardiovascular, and nervous systems. Basically, there is a reason we use words like "gut-wrenching," "heartbreaking," "numb," and "shattered" to describe how grief makes us feel: it can literally do each of these things.

Awesome. Wow.

Which brings me to the week before Adelaide died, when I was sleeping in her bed every night. Not because I needed to, necessarily; she was hooked up to machines that would alert us if anything happened, and we had nurses in our home most nights. But I desperately needed to spend every last moment with her that I could. By that point, we were basically waiting for her to die—it was gut-wrenching and heartbreaking and numbing and shattering. The *only* saving grace of those days was that she was still with us. Other than that, they were basically torture.

One of those horrible, awful, no-good mornings while waiting for her to die, I woke up in her bed, not able to open my eyes. No, I did not have pink eye, and I had not been crying so much that they swelled shut. It was an inflammatory response that would sporadically occur again and again over the following year, each time lasting several days before my eyes would return to some sort of normal—a little faster if I used some of Adelaide's leftover steroids. Was taking my dead daughter's prescription medications a responsible decision? Absolutely not. Did it help? Sure did.

As obvious as it may seem in hindsight, it took me months to realize this was all provoked by my grief and not some ill-timed skin care blunder or new sporadically occurring allergy. But knowing that I hadn't somehow brought it on myself helped. More importantly, though, it pointed me in the right direction: toward a specialist who could do something about it.

Another fun fact: the physical effects from grief are more likely to exacerbate pre-existing conditions.[4] For me, that was skin sensitivity and allergies. With the help of an allergist, I was finally able to get control of these reactions; however, even to this day, if I don't take the right combination of medications, I can feel a burning itch on my eyelids. And I *wasn't* able to find that correct combination before the inflammation response forever changed the shape of my eyes—one now opens a bit less than the other.

These enduring physical effects are just as legitimate and grief-induced as the emotional ones. They are not in our heads and they are not our fault. In fact, as heavy as grief can be, it makes perfect sense that our minds would need our bodies to share the load. Give yourself just as many gold stars for surviving grief's physical effects as you do its emotional ones. And remember that when the world comes calling—your boss, a parent, your child, and they need an email reply, an errand, or breakfast—all you need to do is keep going. Keep surviving one inchstone at a time. Low-hanging fruit is the bar. On better days, we can reach for those higher branches—and one day, you will shock yourself by grasping them.

One day, maybe not today, but someday.

Okay, so I get into this in more detail in chapter five, but writing seriously helped me process my grief. Putting our wildest thoughts and most untenable emotions into words helps contain them. Like putting a leash on a stray dog. They are still a little wild, but you have more control, and in time can even lead them in a more positive direction. Truly, there is *nothing* that helped me more than writing. Still, the last thing I want these after-chapter prompts to feel like is book club fodder (though, if you want to use them that way, by all means do!). Also unlike a book club, no one is going to force you to participate. But should you decide to give it a try, allow your responses to be personal and vulnerable, maybe even a little uncomfortable—I promise I won't share with anyone.

So, at the risk of feeling a little self-help-y: What are some of your weirder impulses that are driven by your grief? Are there ways your grief has affected you physically? What are the simple tasks you enjoy doing that can motivate you to escape the comfort of your bed?

If these prompts don't connect with you, feel free to write about anything that does.

_____

_____

_____

_____

_____

_____

_____

_____

2

When You're Forced into Retirement

> Death ends a life, not a relationship. All the love you
> created is still there. All the memories are still there.
> You live on—in the hearts of everyone you have
> touched and nurtured while you were here.
>
> —Mitch Albom

Until we have lost someone deeply ingrained in the fabric of our lives, it is hard to understand just how life-altering loss can be. One day, they are this central character in your life, and the next they are gone. We miss the individual person, of course. But we also miss the space they took up, the role they played, and how they factored into our daily decisions. Left with vacancies on calendars, daily details longing to be shared, rote routines requiring permanent detours, we are grieving what was once our normal life. We are grieving a piece of our own identity.

Take social media for instance. How many profiles do you come across where someone lists in their bio that they are the proud parent of three and wife to @besthusbandever? How many more list their profession—or a combination of the two: "Dad, husband, teacher, dog lover" or "financial planner by day, child's activity chauffeur by night"? These bios ask us to publicly introduce ourselves to the world and, more often than not, these relationships and titles are what we put out there. It can be nearly impossible to identify ourselves outside of our relationships to others: daughter, grandson, sister, partner, friend, parent, caregiver.

To further complicate matters, these relationships often double as our personal names: on any given day, I am referred to as "Mommy" far more often than "Kelly." In loss, the vision of us the world sees may no longer match how we self-identify. Just last month you were a wife, and in your heart that is still true—but the world now sees a widow. I self-identify as part of a family of five and the mother of three amazing children, even though one has passed away. From the outside, though, we are simply a family of four. People don't see what is missing. They see a single mom but not the joy, love, heartache, and tragedy of her lost spouse. They see a father comforting his child after his son injures himself, but not the man's stinging pain when he realizes that his mother is no longer there to call to ask if he should apply heat or cold to this wound. I'm not saying it's right or wrong to tie our identities to these labels of "wife" or "child" or "dad" or "grandkid." But I want to underline how utterly devastating the loss of one of these titles can be to our self-identity. It can feel as if you've been fired from a job you loved or have been forced into retirement.

I suppose I should have been better prepared for my own forced retirement, considering I had stumbled through several involuntary career changes in the past. The same week Adelaide was diagnosed with epilepsy, my husband Miguel called to tell me he had been offered the title role in the Chicago production of *Hamilton*. Holy humongous detour, Batman! We were living in the New Jersey suburbs, twenty miles outside of New York City, so we could both commute in for work. Years before, I had left my acting career so that we could start a family. At the time, I felt as if I was giving up on my dream and letting childhood Kelly down, but the prospect of two artists trying to support a family in New York City was wildly overwhelming. So I accepted a job working long hours, selling event spaces and coordinating associated events for a restaurant in *Top Chef* judge Tom Colicchio's restaurant group. Turns out, not only did I love the job, I also thoroughly enjoyed having a regular paycheck and fancy health insurance.

Back to that life-changing phone call. Don't get me wrong—I was vibrating with adrenaline-fueled excitement when Miguel shared his incredible news with me, but it didn't take long to see how a cross-country move with a newly-diagnosed-as-disabled daughter was going to drastically effect my career path. My family needed me at home now, to manage this move and eight-month-old Adelaide's complicated health. The sudden loss of my working-mom identity hit hard. In time, I would fall in love with Chicago and with being a fierce advocate for my daughter, but first I had to grieve the life of the financially independent woman that had bought our family's first home and met sales goals like the boss she was.

In a world where basic introductions include the question, "What do you do for a living?" it is no wonder that we tie so much of our identity to our occupation. I know—I'm sure we all know—that our identities are more than our jobs, but knowing that didn't stop me from needing therapy to overcome an emotional breakdown when I left my career to take care of my family. Without my career, who was I? What was my value to my family if it couldn't be determined by a salary contribution?

In hindsight, I can see that this line of thought is clearly ridiculous. But it would take me about a year to grieve my career and not just accept, but own my new job as a stay-at-home mom/nurse/therapist/pharmacist. The rush I got from closing a large sale was replaced by hard-fought advocacy wins on Adelaide's behalf. The value I felt from paying our family's mortgage was replaced by the near-encyclopedic knowledge I collected about my daughter's conditions—knowledge that helped keep her alive. I acknowledged each hole my previous career left in my life and found a way to fill it in my new life.

Again, for context, it took me a year to grieve and adjust from a lost career. One entire year . . . for a career.

Then, with one last strained exhale from my almost-four-year-old daughter's lips, my life once again became utterly unrecognizable. I was forced into retirement from a job I had grown to adore, a job that fulfilled me in ways I never could have imagined when I'd taken it on three years earlier. Sure, our routine was overwhelmingly foreign to most, but it was familiar to me, like an ancient map written in a language only I could translate. It was not a routine I ever would have chosen, but I wasn't exactly consulted on the matter either. After all, who else would have cared for her? Who else would have accepted having their schedule and sleep dictated by her most basic needs, and their self-value tied to how well they met those needs?

I hated that I had to fight for her life, but I loved fighting *for her.*

I hated filling syringes with medicine five times a day, but I loved the knowledge and empowerment that came from caring for her.

I simultaneously hated and loved how much I was needed.

I *was* needed.

And then I wasn't.

"Did you fast before coming in today?" the phlebotomist asked.

"No, but I'm not getting a CMP so it should be fine."

I felt a small adrenaline rush as words came out of my mouth that I hadn't uttered in over a year.

CMP, CBC, VBG—this alphabet soup of blood tests used to be a regular part of my vocabulary, along with words like "quantitative immunoglobulins," "GABAergic," and "fasciculation." It took me years to learn these words, what they meant, and how to read any corresponding test results. But I'd had to if I wanted to be the best caregiver I could be and give Adelaide the best chance at a healthy life.

It hadn't dawned on me until I was sitting in the phlebotomist's chair how much I missed the language and learning that had come with my role. I missed surprising someone with my medical knowledge. I missed being a mama bear and going toe to toe with doctors, discussing and debating what was best for my daughter. I missed that rush that came from knowing I was an expert on Adelaide. No one knew her better.

I realize this may seem bizarre—why would I remember these words and that culture fondly when they caused me and, more importantly, Adelaide so much pain? I get that it could even look ego-driven that I got a rush when advocating for Adelaide. But I would argue that we all feel a rush when we are working, producing, and delivering at our peak. The difference was my job wasn't negotiating a business deal; it was advocating for my daughter.

When Adelaide died, I didn't just lose a person who I loved deeply; I lost a lifestyle, a routine, and a purpose. Who was I if I wasn't Adelaide's mother? If I wasn't the caregiver for a medically complex and disabled child who required my near-constant attention and devotion? How did I spend my time when I wasn't deliberating and preparing for her next doctor appointment, G-tube feed, or seizure? What did I do with all these facts and knowledge neatly filed in my brain for which I now had no practical use? My to-do list had been wiped, but instead of seeing a blank slate, all I saw was the faint outlines of what had once been written there.

Outlines that my most beloved high school teacher, Terry, could relate to. In response to one of my blog posts, he wrote to me about his wife who passed away several years ago.

> *"Everybody complained that Sandy would be so controlling, but the funny thing was that I was the controlling one. She would plan, and I would carry those plans out to the letter. Because of her diabetes I made sure that mealtimes were super specific. I would make sure that I knew exactly where to park that was closest to where we were going . . . When Sandy died, all of a sudden there was no need to plan or control, and I was lost. I don't even think I knew why I was lost, but I was lost. I was pretty much spiraling, and I didn't even know it."*

When a caregiver loses their charge, it is only natural that we feel unmoored, as if we're drifting out to sea under an overcast sky without a map or compass. From the outside looking in, people may suggest or assume that the caregiver-turned-griever finds relief in no longer needing to concern themselves with this multitude of details. But what they saw as a weighted chain was, in fact, our stabilizing anchor.

"How nice that you don't need to check in with the nursing home every day."
"At least you'll never have to coordinate transportation to the clinic again."
"I bet you won't miss those medication alarms going off several times a day!"

There may even be a part of us that *is* relieved to not have these daily concerns. But it's impossible to deny the void left in their wake. Over time, these acts of service became a love language, the way we showed we care and are present. Being forced into retirement leaves us with all the knowledge and love but no clear outlet to express it.

In time, we may find ways to use these hard-earned skills to help ourselves or others, but in the immediate aftermath of loss, there is little we can bear to do aside from pack up our desk in a cardboard box and carry it woefully from the office.

One of life's greatest and most difficult lessons is that we cannot control how people perceive us. Through age and experience, hopefully we can learn to live our lives as true to ourselves as possible, allowing our words and actions to portray our honest selves. I am Kelly first and foremost, but to some little people I am also Mommy, and to my family I am wife, sister, and daughter. These titles and relationships have absolutely molded me into the person I am today. Each of them is a piece of me. But no single relationship is all of me.

I don't say this to minimize how devastating losing any of these titles can be—a piece of you is missing, and we all know that when we look at a puzzle with a missing piece, our eyes are drawn to the hole first. However, the remaining puzzle pieces still make a beautiful picture; we can still appreciate that picture even as we remember the piece that has been lost. Even if the missing piece is not immediately apparent to the outside viewer, its impression is not lost on us, and *that* is what matters. Our memory of the piece and our ability to share that memory is far more important than other people's perception of the completeness of our puzzle. We define our identity, and there is both power and comfort in recognizing that.

In death, there is no going back. Inherently we know this, yet still we cling to what was once normal. Part of being forced into retirement is allowing ourselves time and space to discover our new normal and the new routines that "normal" brings with it. We don't have to like these normals or their corresponding routines at first—we can even resent them for a while—but our repetitive motions will tread fresh paths. This is part of the inevitability of time healing our wounds, whether we want it to or not. Our grief itself will become part of this new normal. It will become part of our ever-evolving identity.

And that's the thing—our identity is *always* evolving. I am not the same person I was twenty years ago (thank goodness). I have not always been a writer or a mother or even in a romantic relationship. Growth, change, and, yes, even loss (especially loss?) add to our layers. Adelaide is no longer my daily responsibility, but I will forever see the world through the glasses of a parent of a medically complex child. Her physical absence can't take away that piece of my lived experience or the titles that once accompanied my relationship with her. Nothing can take any aspect of our identity from us. Our physical circumstances will change, but the impacts that a relationship had on our life are permanent.

We lose so much more than a person when someone dies. Think about all the ways your loss has affected your identity. What are the missing puzzle pieces in your life?

Now, who are you without these missing pieces?

Try writing an introduction to yourself, but leave out your occupation and relationship to others.

If these prompts don't connect with you, feel free to write about anything that does.

_____

_____

_____

_____

_____

_____

_____

_____

_____

_____

_____

_____

3

When You're Grieving the Little Things

Absence diminishes small loves and increases great ones, as the wind blows out the candle and fans the bonfire.

—François VI, duc de La Rochefoucauld

There is so much more to loss than the absence of who or what we adored. To understand our grief is to know that we are grieving more than one strand of vibrantly dyed thread—we are grieving an intricately woven tapestry, and each of those threads must be grieved in their own time.

So. Much. Grief.

Those threads are the food we no longer buy for them at the grocery store, the items we pass by at Target that they would have loved, and the prescriptions that no longer need to be filled. We miss their favorite music, their time-perfected recipes, or their sports team that we cheered on with them. We grieve the plans we made but never realized: a weekend trip to the lake or an extravagant adventure to Paris. Those threads are also the dreams we had together, or that we had for them: graduations, weddings, careers, grandchildren. When you break it all down, it is no wonder that grief is as exhausting and complex as it is. Or why it takes so long to process and can sneak up on us when we least expect it.

I have a framed saying on my desk that reads, "The little things are the big things." A friend gave it to me back when we were fighting for even the tiniest step forward in Adelaide's health and development. Since then, it has taken on new meaning. When I consider the moments I miss most with Adelaide, it isn't her birthday parties or our family trip to Disney World. It is the small moments: snuggling on our couch, reading to her and catching her peeking at the pages. It's the walk around our neighborhood that would calm her when she was crying. It's the way she would squeeze my finger to make sure I was still there.

Being reminded of those seemingly small moments, those single strands of the tapestry we wove with our beloved, especially when the pain is raw and fresh, can be our unraveling. We take out-of-the-way detours to avoid their school, work, or doctor's office. Then the next moment we are clinging to those strands, devouring an entire row of their favorite seasonal Oreos, rereading their favorite book, listening to their favorite song just to feel close to them again. File this under "Grief Is Weird" and just know that you are not alone in this emotional seesaw of the seemingly small stuff.

Sometimes, the weight of these everyday memories can be oppressive, even suffocating, rendering even the most mundane tasks impossible. For example, grocery shopping . . .

I hadn't even reached the threshold of our local supermarket when my hands began to shake. It had been maybe a month since Adelaide died and life was starting to settle into a new normal. Everyone still greeted me with "the look," and it would be months before I slept through the night, but some things (like my family's ability to consume milk, bread, and eggs) would never change. So, here I was, at the store, like I had been thousands of times before. But it felt all wrong. No, *I* felt wrong. Lightheaded, shaky, and clammy, I clung to the grocery cart for stability—was I about to pass out?

I sprinted through the store as if I was on an episode of *Supermarket Sweep,* grabbing only the necessities. The woman who scanned my items at checkout did a poor job of hiding her concern as she eyed my steadying grip on the counter between us, but I didn't care. I just needed to pay and get out of the store. It would take twenty minutes of me sitting in my car, waiting for my heart to slow and my head to clear, before I felt comfortable turning the ignition.

It shouldn't come as a surprise that I relished grocery delivery during the pandemic—and then at some point, I just started delegating food shopping to Miguel. Did he come home with everything on the list? Sure didn't. And, coincidentally, we ended up with more sugar products in our home than ever before. But it was a small price to pay to not have to set foot in a grocery store. In fact, I wouldn't enter a grocery store again for over a year. What's your phobia? Spiders? Germs? Cool, cool, yeah, I don't do grocery stores.

My anxiety had little to do with the store itself and everything to do with all the memories tucked into each aisle, shelf, and display. There were the avocados that we had bought in bulk when Adelaide had been on the ketogenic diet. There was the medicine aisle where I had regularly stocked up on children's Tylenol and suppositories. The diapers, wipes, and baby food that I would never purchase for her again. Everywhere I turned, another memory came rushing at me in the form of produce or dry goods. Combined with the fear of running into someone I knew and having to socialize with them, it was more than I could handle.

"Eventually, you will need to go to the grocery store again," my mother told me.

"Do I though? Between delivery and Miguel, it seems like I've got it covered."

"It's not about the groceries, Kelly. It's about facing your triggers."

Therapeutically adept moms. Ugh.

So, I started with a short list—three items, in and out—and at a grocery store I rarely frequented so that there would be fewer direct memories. I survived. Then I tried the same thing at the grocery store closer to home. In and out, head down, and using self-checkout so I didn't need to speak to anyone. Again, I survived, but this time I was emotionally spent for the rest of the day, barely able to leave the couch. Week after week, I built up my stamina, adding to my list and only going when I felt the most stable.

Here's the thing: we don't have to jump right back into regular life the way we knew it. But we also can't avoid it if we hope to regain any semblance of control. I found ways to take those incremental steps and then give myself space and time afterward to work through it—and it helped. I still don't enjoy grocery shopping and typically delegate it to Miguel (even if the last thing we need is another bag of Sour Patch Kids . . .), but I *can* go. Which, if I must admit it, is the point my mother was trying to make. Going to the grocery should be a choice that's available, not a task to be avoided at all costs. Some days it takes more out of me than others, but it's no longer debilitating. As small a victory as it may seem to do something like go grocery shopping, it's a big deal to me, and I'm pretty freaking proud. Give me all the gold stars!

These small things don't always have to hinder us, though—sometimes they can bring us comfort too. Right next to that framed saying, I have a glass cup filled with markers, pens, pencils, and one syringe. We used to have syringes all over our house—stuffed in between couch cushions, on nightstands, and in coat pockets, purses, and cup holders. Basically, they were as common in our lives as loose change, water glasses, and hair ties: scattered around just where you needed them, and, more often than not, exactly where you didn't.

We used these syringes to give Adelaide her five-times-daily medications, to flush her G-tube after a meal, or to release gas when she was bloated. After each use, they were taken apart, rinsed, laid out to dry, then placed back in their cup by the sink for next time. Such a simple piece of plastic, but these syringes literally kept Adelaide alive. I had my favorites, of course: the ones that the numbers didn't rub off of and the ones with the more durable plastic stoppers. The hospital always had the best ones, so I would ask our nurses to leave me with their used ones instead of tossing them. Then, after Adelaide died, I took the various medical items that had been heaped on the kitchen counter and placed them in her closet.

"Leave the syringes," Miguel said.

So I did. Like a bouquet of clear, plastic flower stems, they sat in the cup in the corner of the kitchen.

In fact, I didn't touch that cup until it was time for us to move from Chicago. In a mindless purging flurry, I threw most of the syringes away, keeping a select few, just because. When we made it to New Jersey and I was unpacking the box of random kitchen utensils that also held the syringes, I was unsure what to do with them. It felt odd to place them back on the counter in a home where they wouldn't be used by a child who would never live there. So, I tucked a couple in a drawer, a few in a medicine cabinet, and then put one in the pencil jar in my office.

Every day that I sit at my desk, I see it. A symbol of the life we once led, it feels right there. Like your childhood blanket at your parent's house.

Of course, Adelaide left behind quite a bit more than a few syringes. Her things, big and small, from her bulky equipment to a misplaced sock, were reminders of her presence and impact on our life. Threads of every size and color that added to my personal grief tapestry.

"I was thinking we could start going through Adelaide's room today," my mom suggested as she made her morning tea. It had only been a few days since Adelaide had passed, though, and it felt wrong and too soon. On the other hand, I appreciated having a task and the help. Mom would only be with us for a few more days before she headed back to North Carolina, and I couldn't imagine sorting through Adelaide's belongings alone—and suffice it to say that Miguel is not the organizing type.

I opened the double doors to Adelaide's closet and stared at the drawers of clothes, baskets of bows, shelves of books, bins of stuffed animals, and scattered medical equipment stuck into every other available nook and cranny. For not having made it to four years old, Adelaide sure had acquired a lot of stuff.

We started with her clothes, sorting the items into piles I wanted to keep and those I would give away, further dividing the giveaway pile among family and dear friends. We chose to put Adelaide's many, many hairbows—except for a few of my favorites—out in a bowl at the reception following her celebration of life service, allowing everyone to take one in her memory. Her extensive stuffed animal and book collections were divided between those with meaning and those without, then boxed up accordingly. All her therapy toys and equipment were gathered and donated to the therapy clinic where she had received services. Then, in the weeks that followed, I would find a service to which I could donate most of her remaining medical supplies.

"What do you want to do with these?" Mom asked, pulling unopened toys and sippy cups from the top back shelf of the closet. It held all items that had been purchased for her before we understood that she would never be able to use them. I had held on to them all, hoping that someday her brain would find peace and we could make developmental progress once again.

"Donate them." Fresh tears fell down tired tracks on my face. "I need a break."

"I'll finish up in here. Why don't you go lay down."

From where I sit now, I am eternally grateful to my mother for initiating that first cleanse of Adelaide's things. The longer I had waited to face that closet, the harder it would have been. The ghosts and memories would have built up, my depression thickening the fog. But in those early days, I was still in shock. I knew her death was real, but we hadn't yet settled into any sort of new normal, and as a result, I was craving productive distraction. When we moved ten months later, I found myself culling her belongings a little more: toys that had been hiding in the bottom of bins, expired medicines tucked away in her cabinet in the kitchen. While a few of her belongings are scattered around our new home as décor, most of her life is now condensed into three plastic tubs. Rarely can I bring myself to open them, but I find comfort knowing they are there.

On occasion I will come across a photo of a friend's daughter wearing a dress or rain jacket that I recognize as Adelaide's. Sometimes they will tag me in the photo letting me know that they are thinking of Adelaide. It hurts seeing another child in these clothes—clothes that once hung on my child. But knowing that her clothes and accessories are being adored and appreciated by people who loved her allows me to feel like a little bit of Adelaide is living on in their families. Recently, when friends have had babies, I've been able to bring myself to open those plastic tubs and find an item of clothing, book, or stuffed animal to gift to their coming child. I know that the item will be cherished far more in their home than it is untouched in my basement.

There is no surefire way to determine what to let go of and what to keep. Knowing how much honor and joy something will bring to someone else helps me part with it—but so does time. I have found that my attachment to certain items has dwindled, and I require the emotional support of her things less than I did. Instead of existing outside my body, her memory has now settled within me. Of course, there are certain items I can't imagine ever parting with: the flower crown my cousin made for her to wear at her last birthday party, pj's she wore that I placed in a ziplock in hopes of preserving her scent. As long as a physical memento still brings me joy, I will hold on to it.

There is no perfect timetable (as long as it happens before you become a candidate for *Hoarders*). If going through their stuff is simply unimaginable right now, then give yourself time. Though as I look around at my many personal memory boxes, clothes, and books, I must admit that I pity the person who must go through *my* belongings when I am gone. Perhaps minimalists are onto something . . . but I could never. Apologies in advance to whoever pulls the short straw on that formidable task.

Sometimes, though, the issue isn't the vast number of things to distribute, store, or part with—it's the lack of mementos. When we lost the pregnancy of our son Elvis (a name my father gave him before Miguel and I had settled on an official name—and then it just kind of stuck) at twenty-one weeks, I grieved the loss of a child that I never got to meet. I had begun to purchase décor for his nursery that we put away in hopes that it would hang in our next baby's nursery, but aside from our ultrasound photos and a few condolence cards, there was nothing else to remember him by. My mother had a wooden memory box carved to hold the few items I did have. As barren as it is, I'm glad to at least have the box. A simple visual placeholder for a life that never was.

Whether it's an overabundance or a scarcity of physical things that you're grappling with, sometimes it helps to remember that not every memento must be from our loved one's life. We can create our own after they have passed. Be it a box, piece of jewelry, or even a tattoo—*we* attach the meaning to physical objects. If you are craving something physical to hold on to, then find or manifest it: have a paving stone dedicated at their favorite stadium, plant a rose bush in your yard, frame a photo. The value in a wedding ring isn't necessarily in the size of the stone (okay, maybe a little bit if it's a really nice one); it is in the love and commitment that the ring symbolizes. Don't have the wedding ring to remember them by because it was lost or maybe there was never a legal marriage? Design your own. We can create value through their memory and in their honor.

A thread of my grief that I found particularly challenging to work through was missing my daughter's people—her nurses, therapists, and medical team. Maybe your person's people are their work colleagues, teammates, friends, or family. These are the people who are still very much alive, but now feel miles away because your main connection to them is gone.

Four days a week, Adelaide's nurse was present in our home. All her attempts to establish and maintain professional boundaries were in vain as I mentally adopted her as a sister. Besides Adelaide, there was no one I spent more time with. She traveled with us to appointments, to therapies, and even on vacation. We chatted about family, relationships, and pets. She was there each morning, ready for the Adelaide care handoff as I switched gears to get Jackson ready for school. And then she wasn't.

Dr. M was Adelaide's epileptologist, and we spoke weekly to discuss changes in her medications as well as new tests or treatments to consider. I sent him research studies I'd found during late-night Google dumpster dives, and encouraged him not to abandon his own research. We would chat about his lovely wife and his son's baseball games, his mother's health and the latest microbrew he had discovered. And then we didn't.

For a while, I questioned whether these friendships were real or just born out of proximity. Without Adelaide, was there even anything to hold us together?

Yes, I decided. There *was*. Adelaide's memory was going to have to be enough of a tether. I adored these people and I needed them in my life. Just as I was navigating and adjusting to other new normals, these relationships could grow and adapt as well. Not *without* Adelaide, but *because* of her.

We had decided to donate a part of Adelaide's brain to science, so I thankfully still had a reason to connect with Dr. M since he had helped facilitate the donation. It was easily one of my most bizarre conversation starters to date, but it was the bridge I needed to make sure that this relationship did not die with Adelaide. He ended up inviting us to his home for dinner, and I got to meet his family who I'd heard so much about. Given my continued advocacy in the epilepsy world, our paths still cross several times a year at conferences and events, and we pick up as if no time has passed.

Maintaining the relationship with Adelaide's nurse was a bit more challenging, due to her more private nature and the fact that she was also deeply grieving Adelaide. After all, she had structured her days around Adelaide for years, just like I had. Even though continuing this relationship has taken more intentionality on my part, there is no question it has been worth it. Several times, when I've been back for visits to Chicago, I've been able to grab a drink with her. We catch up quickly and then usually spend the rest of the time sharing stories and memories about Adelaide. Sometimes there are even stories that I've never heard before or just forgotten. Stories that had me hanging on to every last detail, imprinting them permanently in my memory as if I were experiencing them firsthand. After someone has died, I'm not sure that there is a more precious gift than an untold story or never-before-seen photograph. Rabbi and author Steve Leder wrote, "We lose so much to death. Half our memory is gone with the death of the only person on earth who shared that incredible trip, the pizza from that little place down that alley in Rome, the babies' first stumbles across the room, that old white Ford we took cross country when we were young and had no money."[5] And he's right, to a certain extent. But by maintaining the relationships with the people we had in common, maybe we don't have to lose all of those memories after all, and can even gain some new ones along the way.

I encourage you to not let yourself drift away from these people just because you're no longer tethered to the same dock. It's okay to continue a relationship that you wouldn't have established without your lost loved ones. Go out for coffee, meet up for a drink, attend a game that your loved one would have enjoyed. These relationships will help keep their memory alive *and* give you time with someone who is also grieving. Their grief may look different from yours, but they know what's in your heart, and hopefully they can hold that space with you.

The little things are the big things. They are the traditions, the recipes, and the syringes. They are the people, the sports teams, and the rock bands. Some moments they are our undoing, and in others, they are the threads that bind our pieces together, like that tapestry or, rather, a comforting blanket. Grief is not predictable, and it doesn't always make sense, but neither do life and death. So, give yourself space to respond to the little things as they come, and let how they affect you change over time. Because their effect will change, and so will you.

What is your grocery store? Your syringe? Do they ever trade places?

Is there someone from your person's life who you miss? What would reconnecting with them and that friendship look like? If you're resisting the connection, why? If not, consider this the nudge you need to write that email, send that text, or make that phone call.

If these prompts don't connect with you, feel free to write about anything that does.

* * *

_____

_____

_____

_____

_____

_____

_____

_____

_____

_____

_____

_____

_____

_____

_____

_____

_____

_____

4

When You Realize We All Grieve Differently

Sorrow is so easy to express and yet so hard to tell.

—Joni Mitchell

There are three needs of the griever: To find the words for the loss, to say the words aloud, and to know that the words have been heard.

—Victoria Alexander

My husband is a crier. Animated movies, commercials, dramatic TV shows—you name it, I've caught him snotting and sniffling through it. Yet, when our daughter died, *our daughter*, his tears were sparse.

It's not that he didn't cry at all—he was Waterworks McGee at the beginning—but as the days became weeks and then months, I couldn't remember the last time I had seen him emotionally affected in any obvious or visible way by our loss. Meanwhile, I was still crying myself to sleep in our daughter's bed and sobbing with abandon on our bathroom floor. Why was I the only one grieving her still? Was there something wrong with me? I already felt so alone in my grief, and here was the one person, the *only* person, who truly understood this specific loss—and his grief was nowhere to be seen. I had heard over and over again that everyone grieves differently, but until then I hadn't understood how difficult grieving differently would be.

After a suggestion from my mother, I made an appointment with a couples' counselor. My relationship with Miguel felt strong in every other way, but I also knew that marriages had crumbled from far less than child loss. I had been a frequent client of mental health professionals since I began visiting the school counselor in third grade following the death of my grandmother. In the years since that loss, I've spent more time in therapy than not. Conversely, Miguel was a therapy rookie. I wasn't sure what would come of it, but it just felt like the right thing to do.

Sitting in the therapist's leather-bound office, it didn't take long for the conversation to steer toward how differently Miguel and I were grieving. When the therapist asked Miguel what he does when he hears me crying in the bathroom, Miguel answered that he doesn't do anything because he figures I want to be alone.

"Kelly, is that what you want?" asked the therapist.

"Maybe initially, but then I just want a hug and to know that I'm not alone in feeling all of this. Grief is already lonely, but to feel like I'm the only one grieving in my own house is maddening." The therapist passed me a box of tissues to dry the tears now pouring from my face. "I wish you would meet me in the dark places with your grief," I said, now facing Miguel.

Miguel stared at his clasped hands where they rested in his lap in response.

"Miguel, is there a reason you keep your grief from Kelly?"

"I don't know, I just prefer to grieve alone. I *am* grieving—it's just at night when everyone is asleep." He paused to gather his thoughts. Or maybe his courage. "I also don't feel like I have the right to grieve Adelaide as much as Kelly does. I feel guilty that I wasn't around as much. My grief isn't the same."

Maybe this therapist was amazing, or Miguel was a therapy prodigy, but either way, I was stunned into silence. First, by the poignant pain of

Miguel's admission, and then because he had realized and admitted this in a single session.

In the 1990s, researchers Kenneth Doka and Terry Martin set out to determine the differences between the way men and women grieve. In their book, *Men Don't Cry, Women Do,*[6] they concluded that, while women are more likely to grieve in one way and men another, it is nowhere near universal. They would go on to revise their findings in their 2010 book, *Grieving Beyond Gender,*[7] where they acknowledge that grief is best understood on a spectrum. At one end of that spectrum is what they referred to as "intuitive" grieving, with "instrumental" grieving on the other. Gender can play a role in the way we grieve, but it is only one of many factors.

Intuitive grievers are the more emotional types who are going to feel *all* their emotions: love hard, grieve hard. These are the snot-faced, puffy-eyed, can't-stop-crying-in-public folks who just need to sit in their well of grief until it has dried up and they can slowly re-enter the light. Instrumental grievers are far more likely to internalize their grief, to intellectualize and rationalize it. Their grief will not be as visually apparent, but is no less significant.

But even this spectrum does not encapsulate all types of grief. Doka and Martin also acknowledge dissonant grief, which occurs when someone has a difficult time expressing on the outside the way they are feeling their grief on the inside. This can go both ways. It may be due to cultural or societal pressures that tell them they cannot, or *should* not, express their true emotions. Or maybe they slather on the guilt because they do not feel as broken up as they think they should, and as a result feel their visible grief feels performative. Was that what Miguel was experiencing? I believe that Miguel was internally broken up *enough* (whatever "enough" is), but I do know that, in general, he often struggles with emotion feeling performative—perhaps that's the cost of doing business as an actor. Throw in some guilt, and I can certainly see how that could breed moments of dissonant grief.

Now that our technical definitions are out of the way, I should note that I generally despise labels (how dare someone try to pigeonhole me into being one specific type of person!). I am in control of who I choose to be and will not be predestined to respond because some researcher said it would be so. That said, I *love* a good spectrum. While labels can feel constrictive in an all-or-nothing kind of way, a spectrum provides some individualized fluidity that I can identify with and proactively use to better understand both myself and others.

On this spectrum, I lean more heavily toward the intuitive grieving side. While I may suppress my emotions for a short while, that likely means the impending grief-plosion will be that much more virulent. Then, when the fog has lifted and I'm capable of rational thought again, I will process what led up to my emotive eruption. Be it through free-writing or just sitting with my own thoughts, undistracted by screens or people, I can take steps toward processing what I'm feeling. However, like a good instrumental griever, I also enjoy turning my grief into something productive: fundraising for causes in Adelaide's honor and, well, writing a book.

On the other hand, Miguel—while he still needs to express his grief—does so in a much more controlled manner at convenient times of his choosing. He spends far more time in a rational state of mind than an emotional one, assessing positives and negatives, and problem-solving. Which, to anyone outside his heart and mind, looks like he isn't thinking of his loss at all. Interestingly, while he is happy to channel his grief into something productive—as a traditional instrumental archetype would—he will not be the one to kick-start or spearhead a fundraiser or nonprofit in Adelaide's honor (perhaps that's the dissonance coming through?). He will, though, happily participate.

When it comes down to it, though, I believe that our place on this spectrum is fluid. We may be more intuitive one day and instrumental the next. Or maybe, as we process our grief, we may gradually slide closer to a different end of the spectrum than we started on. Nothing about grief is fixed, so it tracks that neither is the way we choose to express it.

Other factors are at play as well. For example, Miguel's early grief was softened by a relief and acceptance that I still struggle to achieve. In his own words:

"I yell at my son when he forgets to look for traffic on his bike. I have watched tears well up in his eyes as I scold him. I don't do this to scare him or out of anger. I do this because it is my job to protect him. To do everything I can to prevent him from experiencing pain or harm.

I watched my daughter suffer.

I heard her scream.

I saw her body betray her.

I could not scold her. "Stop doing that or you'll get hurt!!!"

I could not protect her. So, when she died I felt calm. I felt relief. I felt unimaginable sadness and pain of my own. But for her, I felt peace. That was everything I had ever wanted for her during her short life."

To be clear, Miguel didn't want her to die or think that death was in some way better for her than her life with disabilities—that would be ludicrous. What he recognized was that we had exhausted all available treatments and, still, her body was dying, still, she was suffering. Miguel was light-years ahead of me here. I had only *just* accepted that there was nothing else we could do to help her when we entered hospice a few weeks before she passed. Of course, I never wanted her to feel pain and hated that I couldn't protect her from it during her life—but it was a cold comfort that her death brought that peace, even if it was rationally true.

When Adelaide had been first diagnosed, our experiences were in lockstep. But we had started this next phase of our grief journey from entirely different places, so it only makes sense that we would express our grief differently.

The most important takeaway here is that there is no right or wrong way to grieve. Doka and Martin acknowledge that both the intuitive and instrumental grieving types are capable of healthy healing, which, according to them, is the ability to reach and accept new types of normal. The path to get to normal is just different for each person as they occupy their own—*variable*—place between intuitive and instrumental grief.

When multiple people are grieving the same loss in different ways but still need each other for support, what do you do? Miguel's and my grieving disparities caught me so off guard because this wasn't even close to the first time we'd grieved during our marriage. Heck, we had been grieving the life we thought we were going to have with Adelaide since her first seizure when she was seven months old. The difference was that then there had been exceedingly little time to be emotional: there were children to care for; medications, therapies, and appointments to manage; various *Hamilton* events; and then regular life mixed in. During Adelaide's life, Miguel and I would check in with each other at least once a week. It was typically in bed on one of his nights off. We would make sure our minds were in agreement on medical decisions and our hearts were in sync about everything else. I guess we were both leaning toward the instrumental end of the spectrum out of necessity.

But now, without the minute-to-minute preoccupation with Adelaide's health and well-being, I had drifted more toward my natural state on the intuitive end. And this is about the time that I realized Miguel and I weren't checking in with each other the way we used to. That is, until we were forced to while sitting in front of a stranger. Perhaps the breakthrough happened because we were paying the therapist and didn't want to waste our money, or, more likely, because we care about each other and didn't want to lose what we had fought for years to maintain. Regardless, we reestablished our weekly emotional check-ins.

"I understand you prefer to grieve alone, and I can respect that, but is it possible to let me know afterward? Maybe that's awkward, but it would be helpful to know that I'm not the only one that gets emotional," I asked Miguel. We were back in our safe space, lying next to each other in our bed, in the dark.

"I can try," Miguel promised, rolling on to his side to look at me. "And when you are having a moment, I'll do a better job of checking on you, but I need you to tell me if you want me to stay with you or you want time alone."

"I can do that."

These asymmetrical grief responses don't just affect romantic relationships. For example, you also spend your entire life with various members of your family, but that doesn't mean that you are going to inherently know or understand how they are grieving. Some people will want or even need a place setting left at the holiday table for the loved one who's passed, while other members of the same family will see this as a twist of a knife. We must open these dialogues to discuss what we are feeling, how we are feeling it, and how we can communicate for everyone to exist in their new normals in the healthiest way possible. A daughter is going to grieve her mother far differently than her father grieves his wife. Even siblings will grieve differently because they each had their own unique relationship with their lost loved one. Different isn't wrong, and it isn't a competition, it just is. Actress Ashley Judd put it beautifully when she said, about grieving for her mother, "We don't have to be congruent in order to have compassion for each other."[8]

Even when you communicate compassionately, though, the person who you thought would be your primary support may still not be able to fill that role in the way you need them to. Perhaps they are the person you are grieving, or the same loss also consumes them, or, for their own personal reasons, they have difficulty connecting with you on this loss. It's okay to turn to someone new, to outsource the comfort and support they once provided you. Just because Miguel wasn't going to ugly-cry with me didn't mean that there weren't other people in my life who would. It also didn't mean that our relationship was doomed. It just meant that for this specific, expansive, and *momentarily* all-consuming part of my life, he wasn't always able to help me the way I was used to.

But as the one-year anniversary of Adelaide's death crept closer, I grew increasingly anxious about how the day would affect my marriage. Like toddlers on a play date, content to engage side by side in parallel play, Miguel and I had fallen into a practice of parallel grieving. We were working toward a feasible blend of our varied grieving styles that was manageable in our everyday life, but an anniversary of this magnitude was far from everyday. I knew he wouldn't be able to be there for me the way I needed, or the way I wished we could be for each other. So, instead of fighting it, instead of setting myself up for epic and preventable disappointment, I called in reinforcements: our best friends from Chicago.

"Do you drink the tap water here or should I get it from the fridge?" Jenny asked me.

"Either is fine, or you can ask Miguel to explain his kitchen counter water filtration system to you."

Miguel had tested our tap water and discovered it had an exorbitant amount of extra stuff in it. So he'd devised a double filtration system that now sat on the counter next to the sink. It was essentially just a combination of store-bought water filters, but he had a system for filter rotation that I never bothered to pay attention to, let alone adhere to, and instead got my water from the tap, which left Miguel exasperated.

"It's not that complicated. When one filter is nearing the end of its life, I switch it out for a new filter and use the old one as the second filter to make sure we get as much stuff out of the water as possible. It tastes so much better—just try it," Miguel urged.

"Wait, so which pitcher am I supposed to drink from? And do I need to switch the filters myself? How often do you have to refill the first pitcher?" Jenny asked Miguel, grinning as she turned to get less complicated water from the fridge.

On Adelaide's deathiversary, while our children played, Jenny, her husband, Miguel, and I watched old episodes of *Schitt's Creek* and laughed at their family's shenanigans, much the same way we had during Adelaide's last weeks when I was desperate for distraction. Toward the end of the evening, I escaped upstairs to our bedroom for a tear-fueled grief exorcism, and then continued laying in bed, unable to stop the now silent stream of tears. After about ten minutes, Jenny quietly lay down in bed next to me. With an arm around me, she lay crying too, both of us just missing Adelaide together.

When she sensed my tears were slowing, Jenny broke the silence. "I have a question, though," she said.

"Okay . . ."

"Can you please try to explain to me how I'm supposed to get a glass of water in your house?"

I snorted as my tears turned to laughter, and Jenny cackled beside me.

This was what I needed in this moment: someone to sit in the dark with me and then shine a light on a way out. This was what Miguel was unable to do for me, or with me, at his own stage of grief. After several more minutes of loving jokes at Miguel's expense, we made our way back downstairs to our children and husbands, and I survived the remaining hours of the day.

Instead of dwelling on how your person isn't helping, turn to someone who can. When your friends tell you to call them whenever you need to talk or cry, take them up on it! After all, if your person-in-chief didn't know how to fix a broken pipe, you wouldn't get mad at them—you would call a plumber. Likewise, if your go-to person cannot fill one of your social or grieving needs, there is nothing wrong with outsourcing it to someone who can.

"How did you sleep?" I asked Miguel as he came downstairs, months later, target-locked on the coffee pot.

"Okay, I guess. I was trying to finish grouting the shower last night, and I began thinking about what it would be like if Adelaide lived here with us. So, I just sat there crying as I lay the grout lines thinking about her and this new house." He was focused on making his coffee while he was telling me this, as if he was just chatting about a tile that wouldn't lay right. But it was so much more than that, and we both knew it.

"I love you. Thank you." I pulled his body around to give him a proper hug. His simple admission meant the world to me. For a moment, I felt less lonely, and our relationship felt more connected.

Just because our preferred tools of the grief trade differ doesn't mean we can't still build and progress on our grief journey together. However, this would never have happened if we hadn't discussed how we preferred to grieve and what we needed emotionally in front of a perfect stranger. Maybe you don't need a (professional) stranger to mediate your conversation, but we all need to have these conversations with the people closest to us.

If you've ever watched a workout video, you may notice that they often have one person doing a beginner version of the exercise and someone else doing a more advanced version. For my friends who aren't quite ready to wrap their legs around their head yet, forget the grieving spectrum for a moment: What are your most basic needs as a griever? What support do you wish you had?

And for my more bendy friends: After identifying your needs and where you sit on the spectrum (if that's even helpful to you), where can each of these needs be met? What resources are available to you, and how can you access them?

If these prompts don't connect with you, feel free to write about anything that does.

_____

_____

_____

_____

_____

_____

_____

_____

_____

_____

_____

_____

5

When the Voice in the Back of Your Head Won't Shut Up

Guilt is perhaps the most painful companion of death.
—Elisabeth Kübler-Ross

At some point during puberty, most of us develop a little voice in the back of our heads that whispers salty negative nothings. Ideally, as you get older, you learn to ignore that voice, or at least turn down the volume a bit . . . and then you hold your child for the first time and it all goes to hell. That voice, which you've trained your entire adult life to tune out, is now blasting at an eleven.

How did I let myself live in denial for so long?

*If I'd been home instead of working, would
I have noticed the seizures sooner?*

Still, I'm a fairly confident person and learned to tune out my inner negative voice not long after Jackson was born. But with Adelaide and all her medical complexities, the voice not only didn't go away—it got louder and more persistent. This difference shouldn't seem all that earth-shattering. After all, the parenting decisions I made with Jackson were more common: Breast milk or formula? Public or private school? But the decisions I made on a daily basis for Adelaide were life or death.

We should have spent more time doing her physical therapies.

She loved going on walks, why didn't we go on more walks?

During Adelaide's life, nearly everyone I met, from relatives to strangers on the internet, had ideas or opinions on how to improve her condition. *Have you tried this brand of essential oils? CBD oil? This special therapy that's exclusively available in upstate New York? I'm sure she'll grow out of it. She doesn't look that sick.* And on and on.

We should have tried a different combination of meds.

What if we had pushed harder for brain surgery?

In the early days, I latched on to every suggestion, every idea with the strength of a thirty-foot-long anaconda. My Google dumpster dives went so deep I needed an oxygen tank. But in time, as my knowledge about her conditions grew and I gathered a medical team that my family trusted, I found a confidence in our decisions that allowed me to drown out the opinions of anyone who was not a part of her inner care circle. Unless someone had taken the time to sit down and go through the hundreds of pages of medical charts, notes, and test results or they had spent significant time with her attempting to understand her ever-fluid physical and cognitive baseline—well, unless that happened, not to be horribly blunt, but their thoughts and opinions were irrelevant. So, if I could eventually drown out other people's voices, there must be a lesson in there somewhere that could teach me to drown out my own . . . right? The problem, I found, was that my inner backseat driver was louder than all of the external noise put together.

What if we stopped fighting too soon?

What if we were forcing her to suffer by keeping her alive?

Sometimes the voice was ignited by an article or social media post I read. But, more often than not, I would be doing something mundane, like folding laundry or helping Jackson with homework, when the whispers would slither up from my subconscious. By the time Adelaide passed away, I had gotten so used to the voice's nagging presence that it seemed totally natural for it to hang around.

This voice is just one symptom of a larger issue: guilt. Grief and guilt go hand in hand. Guilt for not having done more, guilt for neglecting others while you *were* doing more. Guilt for feeling relieved that the struggle is over and guilt when recognizing that there are so many others still struggling. Guilt for falling short on your responsibilities when your grief is debilitating and guilt for being short with people you care about when grief has exhausted your inhibitions. Guilt for laughing. Guilt for finding peace. Guilt for living. Guilt for surviving.

Ah, survivor guilt. I had previously thought of survivor guilt as simply feeling guilty that someone else had suffered and you did not. Like when you're the lone survivor of a plane crash, or your sibling takes the blame when you *both* forgot to feed the dog (who subsequently ate the legs off the couch). But it actually encompasses much more than that. While survivor guilt is not something you can be officially diagnosed with (yet), psychologist Dr. Ellen Hendriksen writes in a 2017 article that survivor guilt is closely associated with PTSD (which *is* an official diagnosis) and all its accompanying symptoms: avoidance and feeling on edge, vigilant, detached, and easily startled. But, she writes, "PTSD-like symptoms aren't the only signs of survivor['s] guilt. Additional signs include obsessing over what happened, feeling confused, unworthy, or ambivalent about living, harping on the meaning of life, or being plagued by the sense that no matter where you go, you're never really safe."[9]

The American Psychological Association describes survivor guilt as "a common reaction stemming in part from a feeling of having failed to do enough to prevent the event or to save those who did not survive . . . or by family or friends who feel that they did not do enough to succor their loved ones prior to death."[10]

In addition to showing me that we do not use the word "succor" enough, my new understanding of survivor guilt inspired me to reach out to a few friends to see what their tricks were for managing their guilt. Most were as lost as me, but one shared that she had named the voice in her head. Personifying the voices allowed her to direct her frustration and resistance *at* something, all while stripping the thoughts of their alien and amorphous qualities, the same way Velma, Daphne, and Fred (and Scooby and Shaggy, too, if only by accident) unmask the monster that's been chasing them. *Aw shucks, it's not a seven-foot-tall tentacled monster; it's just Jasper the groundskeeper!* The more we turn our inner voice into just a Jasper or [insert your own name choice here], the less power we give it. This doesn't mean we instantaneously return to our less-affected selves, just that it can help us have a more positive and healthier outlook on life. Which is how I came to name mine Audrey III.

Between Miguel's work schedule, which meant he was rarely home in the evenings, and Adelaide's demanding nighttime medication routine, Jackson had missed out on experiencing traditional family movie nights. The year after Adelaide died—particularly in those early days of the pandemic when people had not yet tired of Zoom happy hours and jigsaw puzzles were all the rage, when Broadway theaters were dark and Adelaide's medications were tucked away in a cabinet—Miguel and I took the opportunity to introduce Jackson to a few cinematic classics.

The Sound of Music, Annie, and *Newsies* were interspersed with *Back to the Future, Indiana Jones,* and *Ghostbusters.* Jackson would grumble about the graphics or quality of the films, but he gave away his enjoyment when he'd inquire about the next movie during breakfast each day. In the evenings, snuggled on our couch under blankets, we sang along and shared our own childhood memories of these movies in a modern-day Norman Rockwell kind of way.

"What are we watching tonight?" Jackson asked.

"How about *Little Shop of Horrors*?" I suggested.

Jackson's eyes got big. "Is it scary?"

"Nah, it's a musical about a plant that eats people! . . . But not in, like, a scary way. It's funny," Miguel said.

Jackson looked at us in disbelief, with one eyebrow raised (an expression I had taught him), but he ultimately caved. Cuddled up, we watched as the poor plant-shop worker, Seymour, discovers a strange plant, which he names Audrey II (after his crush, Audrey), and incidentally learns of its cravings for blood. What begins as Seymour feeding Audrey II droplets of blood from his pricked finger devolves into campy horror as Audrey II grows and becomes meaner, more demanding, and, well, musical.

Poor Seymour. Can you even imagine living, every day, with an evil voice constantly second-guessing you and demanding to be fed?

Why yes, yes I can.

I should have tried harder to get her into that study. What if the next doctor would have had the answers? These thoughts, like Audrey II, grew louder and more persistent the more time and energy I gave them. I knew they were unhelpful at best and harmful at worst, but I couldn't figure out how to make them go away. Nor, to be honest, did I believe I deserved to have them go away. Part of me accepted them as my penance for surviving when Adelaide didn't, for not being able to save her, for the unimaginable suffering she endured while all I could do was look on and hold her.

The rational side of my brain would try to step up and shout back: *Stop should-ing yourself! What-ifs won't help you heal!*—which is true, but these simple clichés glanced off Audrey III's vines with little effect. If I truly wanted to silence my singing plant monster, or at least hit mute for a little while, I would need to ground myself in stronger and deeper rational truths. The kind that form the physical laws of the universe as we know it. I would have to hit pause on my downward spiral and ask myself a few simple questions.

- Can I travel back in time?
- Did I make the best decision with the information I had at the time?
- Am I psychic?

Let's start with time travel. Barring the existence of some super-classified time machine in a heavily protected bunker in the middle of the desert somewhere, the answer to this question is a resounding no. So, if I can't go back in time, if no positive action can be taken today to change the past, then why am

I spending time and valuable energy contemplating my Guilt Monster's slanderous questions or accusations? Beating myself up over a decision we made and acted upon will not bring Adelaide back to me. It doesn't make me a better or worse person, mother, wife, or friend, and it certainly doesn't help me feel better·or move forward.

In fact, I would argue that dwelling on these past shoulda, woulda, couldas doesn't allow us to be present in our current life, meaning we risk making similar perceived errors in judgment and wishing we had yet another time machine. Our energy is finite, and if we are spending significant brainpower beating ourselves up over the past, then we're pulling focus from what is directly in front of us. Remaining so focused on our past that we miss out on the present can create a vicious cycle of regret. If we're going to think about all the things we wish we would have done differently, then the least we can do is try to learn from these supposed mistakes so we do not repeat them. Rather than stewing, let's just acknowledge these shoulda, woulda, couldas; recognize we cannot change the past; take whatever lesson they are offering; and then move on.

Now that we've established that we can't time travel, let's cut ourselves some slack by coloring in our memories with context. Specifically, did I make the best decision with the information I had at the time?

Adelaide was only two years old when her pulmonologist first told me she would require additional oxygen if we were going to bring her on a plane. Adelaide had a cold, and he was concerned about her maintaining her oxygen levels. I was annoyed because traveling with Adelaide was already challenging. Between her medications, supplies, specialized food, and basic baby needs, my father said we looked like we were traveling with a small rock band. Additionally, Adelaide often screamed on flights—like, the entire flight—and would have the occasional seizure, you know, just for fun. And now we were adding a portable oxygen concentrator.

But you know what? She never screamed or had a seizure on a plane again. Turns out all that screaming and those seizures were because she hadn't been able to maintain her oxygen levels on planes for some time. There is a picture I texted to my parents of me holding Adelaide on a plane, while she is screaming and I'm making a "please help me" face. Whenever I come across the photo, I can feel Audrey III's vines tightening around my chest as the guilt takes over. Here I was taking a photo to make light of this terrible situation, and meanwhile my daughter was literally crying for more oxygen.

But I didn't know that at the time.

When we look back on our past actions, we are able to do so with the . . . gift . . . of hindsight, and let me tell you, perspective is a messy bitch. Just because you can look back at these situations as the person you are now, that doesn't mean you should. You have to look back as the person you were then. The hope is that you can eventually acknowledge that you did the absolute best under the circumstances and with the knowledge you had *at the time*. You can't punish past you because of information only future you has access to.

Next up: Am I psychic? This one is useful when Audrey III is spitting out thoughts like, *We really should have taken that trip together. If only I hadn't worked late that night.* Or, *why didn't I see the symptoms sooner?* When Adelaide was born, there were a handful of tiny red flags that went up: she had poor head control, trouble maintaining her weight, and coughed a lot when I was nursing her. But I didn't want to overreact—whatever was going on, I was sure she would grow out of it. But she wasn't growing out of it, and then the diagnoses started rolling in: hypotonia, developmental delays, generalized epilepsy. Still, I tried desperately to cling to optimistic denial. Then infantile spasms—a developmentally devastating form of pediatric epilepsy—were thrown into the mix. Because of Adelaide's low muscle tone, they only showed as a slight head bob. How long had she been doing that? Days? Weeks? Why hadn't I raised the alarm? How much damage had already been done? If we had caught it sooner, could we have prevented future suffering?

These ulcer-inducing questions are totally unfair. I didn't see these symptoms because I didn't know to look for them. You didn't take the vacation because you thought you would have a lifetime of vacations to look forward to, or money was tight, or you were tired, or there were too many obligations at home. You worked late that night because you *aren't clairvoyant*. You didn't know what you didn't know, and none of us can see into the future. So cut yourself some slack and tell your Audrey III to can it.

Every question in this chapter is one that I have wrestled with repeatedly, asking myself if any of it would have made a difference in Adelaide's quality or length of life. If my self-inflicted emotional wounds were physical, I would be covered in bruises and have several broken bones. But to what end? The actual answers to my Guilt Monster's questions are irrelevant. If life was a Choose Your Own Adventure book and I could flip-flop around looking at my options, then perhaps second-guessing myself in these ways would be productive. But it's not.

I cannot change the past.

I did the best I could in the moment.

I am not psychic.

It is also worth stressing that our guilt is not inherently evil, even if I do often refer to it as a monster. Or, maybe, rather, it's a necessary evil. It is our fear of feeling guilt that provides the lane bumpers we need to be kind, compassionate, and conscientious humans. Lowercase-g guilt is useful. Capital-G Guilt Monsters are not. Unfortunately, shrinking our capital-G Guilt Monster down to basic-g guilt will take more than personification and a few basic questions.

"Okay, you've seen the newest Star Wars movies, but I don't think you've seen the originals," I said to Jackson while washing the dishes after dinner one night.

"With Darth Vader and light savers?" Jackson asked.

"Light SABERS, and yes," I corrected.

Miguel imitated a mechanical breathing sound with one hand over his mouth as he brought me dishes from the dining table, "'Luke, I am your father.'"

"Did you know Darth Vader doesn't actually say that?" I asked.

Miguel looked at me in disbelief. "What?!"

"He says, 'No, *I* am your father.'" I responded.

"Huh, who knew?"

"The internet . . ." Jackson quipped as he settled in on the couch.

I half expected Jackson to be thoroughly unimpressed by the antiquated special effects of the galaxy far, far away, but even in the age of green screens and computer animation, the movies held their own. So did the concept of the dark side.

Yoda: *Yes, a Jedi's strength flows from the Force. But beware of the dark side. Anger, fear, aggression; the dark side of the Force are they. Easily they flow, quick to join you in a fight. If once you start down the dark path, forever will it dominate your destiny, consume you it will, as it did Obi-Wan's apprentice.*

Luke: *Vader . . . Is the dark side stronger?*

Yoda: *No, no, no. Quicker, easier, more seductive.*

Quicker, easier, and more seductive indeed. If our Guilt Monster is the personification of our guilt and doubt, then our Dark Side is its overlord. It is the ultimate manifestation of our combined trauma, guilt, and grief. It is with the Dark Side that we attempt, often in vain, to grasp at a reason why such horrible things happened to us or someone we love—to place blame and attempt to protect ourselves from this pain occurring again.

To resist the pull of my Dark Side would require some seriously strong weaponry—so maybe Jackson was right; maybe it was a light *saver* that we needed after all. But how do you battle against thoughts and ideas? To wound something infinite, I would need a weapon that was equally limitless. What I didn't realize is that I had been brandishing my light saver long before I recognized its power.

Through my journals and blogs, I had been using words and language to beat back the darkness all along. With this awareness, combined with a more directed intention, the effectiveness of my writing grew tenfold. The more I got my thoughts out of my head and into the world, the better I felt. Be that through writing or talk therapy, my thoughts were far less scary when they were defined by words. Words trap our irrational thoughts and force them to materialize into something we can rationally address, analyze, and poke holes in. Consider all the times you've said or heard someone say, "Sorry, that sounded ridiculous out loud," or "That sounded scarier in my head." Like a grinding stone, words smooth our Dark Sides' jagged edges.

In the deep, dark space of our minds, where our most lawless and frightening thoughts rule the land, language is a griever's powerful ally. Those unruly thoughts, when confined to letters, words, and sentences, transform even the most fearsome bad guy into a benign presence.

As the daughter of a mental health therapist, I would be remiss not to encourage you to speak to someone professionally. Friends and family are great, but they bring their own guilt and biases to the conversation. A therapist will help to sort out the rational thoughts from the irrational ones—and if they upset you with a revelation, then at least you don't have to sit across from them at the Thanksgiving dinner table!

We also live in the golden age of psych meds. (Woo hoo!) There is nothing weak about needing medication. Perhaps your anxiety or depression is situational and you only need the pills for a little while. Or maybe, like me, you will need to be on them for the rest of your life. That's fine. If the doctor told you to take a blood pressure medicine, you wouldn't tell them "No, I'm strong enough to manipulate my blood pressure through sheer force of will." Well, we're also not strong enough to manipulate the chemical reactions occurring in our brains, especially during times of great stress and grief.

My mother, the therapist, would also like to stress that it's important to see a *psychiatrist* for psych meds whenever possible. While many primary care physicians and even ob-gyns will prescribe anti-anxiety or anti-depressant medication, psychiatrists are most familiar with the best medications, possible side effects, and proper dosing. And if a medication doesn't seem to work, that doesn't mean that all medications aren't for you. It just means that either the dose wasn't right or you need to try a different medication—which are things that a psychiatrist is better equipped to help with than any other doctor.

By no means am I hawking pills over here, but I've learned that grief is a *journey*. So, consider hiring a guide and picking up a few thoughtfully prescribed supplies to help make that trip, if not easier, at least a little more navigable. The road is long and the path can be arduous, but if you can find any way to shrink your Guilt Monster, then that's much less weight to carry.

What does your Guilt Monster look like, smell like? What is its name? What questions does it hurl at you most often?

Now, using your light saver, aka your writing instrument of choice, how do you respond? Or, perhaps ultimately even more helpfully, why do you choose not to respond?

If these prompts don't connect with you, feel free to write about anything that does.

⇢⇢⇢⟩⟩⟩⟩⟩⇠

_____

_____

_____

_____

_____

_____

_____

_____

_____

_____

_____

_____

_____

_____

_____

_____

6

When Ready or Not, Here Comes Change

> Nothing is so painful to the human mind as a great and sudden change.
>
> —Mary Shelley

Change is inevitable. In many ways, so is our resistance to it, even when the change in question *isn't* monumentally life-altering. Google "resistance to change grief," and four of the first six articles are written for business managers trying to help their employees adapt to change within their company. But whether it's losing a person or an organizational shake-up, humans just aren't great at change—and it doesn't help that grief resulting from the loss of a loved one creates not just one change, but a cascading series of them.

First there is the epic change of our person no longer being in our life, which results in additional major life changes, like what to do with their things, which then sparks even more loss and grief. Life's insistence on moving forward and changing without our permission powers all of this to the nth degree.

Sometimes it can feel like we're stuck on a runaway train and other times like we are being left behind.

The consensus of those aforementioned business articles is to utilize the Kübler-Ross Change Curve—the model for stages of grief developed by Elisabeth Kübler-Ross. Initially, she defined five stages, but those eventually grew to seven: shock, denial, anger, bargaining, depression, acceptance, and processing. There are plenty of books out there that dive into each of these grieving stages, so I'll spare you. And, frankly, I get frustrated with the stages because the way they are typically presented makes it feel like we are somehow supposed to move through them linearly. Folks would ask me which grieving stage I was currently in, and all I could picture were steps on a staircase where, once you climb to "acceptance" and "processing," you are magically cured of your grief by a ray of golden shining light or aliens or something. But grief isn't linear, so if I'm moving backward, forward, and diagonally through these neat, straightforward stages, does that mean I'm failing at grief? Because my inner perfectionist can't handle that.

The thing is, Kübler-Ross herself said that the stages are, in fact, nonlinear.[11] Which makes the question, "How far along are you in your grief?" illogical. (I'm not failing at grieving! It's just not like that!) All anyone can report is what stage they are in at this very moment of this very day, because it can change five minutes from now, leaving the griever in *any* of the six other stages. While the grieving stages have not been super helpful for me on a grander scale, when I look at smaller pieces of my grief, specifically how I handled change while grieving, or handled change that occurred as a result of my grief, these stages have allowed me to better understand how the changes affect me, as well as my reactions to them. This doesn't make me less of a mess in the moment, but hopefully brings clarity afterward, which I can use to better prepare for future changes. First, though, comes the mess, as I would so perfectly demonstrate when we made the bittersweet move from Chicago to New Jersey.

All are welcome to attend a Celebration of Life for Adelaide Grace Cervantes in your most colorful attire, the invitation read.

It had been my mother's idea to call it a celebration of life and to have everyone dress in color instead of black. I definitely wasn't in the mood to "celebrate," but went along with it because I figured acknowledging the death of a child was excruciating enough. If we could brighten the day with color and semantics, then why the hell not.

An army of friends, family, and colleagues descended on us from across the country to help us put the best possible day together, but there were still a few personal touches that I wanted to take care of myself. So, my first trip out of the house following Adelaide's death was to a craft store to pick up picture frames, baskets, and a guest book for the service. Miguel and his brother dropped off my mom and me before heading to Target with their own list. As I walked the aisles, my peripheral vision dulled, and all I saw was whatever was directly in front of me. I'm sure there were other people in the store with us, but I don't remember seeing any.

As we stood in the store's vestibule waiting for Miguel to return, I let myself fall into a daze, watching the rain hit the glass windows. Octobers in Chicago often stayed warm until days before Halloween, but that day there was a telling chill in the air, accompanied by fog and a heavy drizzle— undoubtedly an appropriate backdrop for the day. When our minivan rolled up with Adelaide's handicap placard still hanging from the rearview mirror, Mom and I ran to the car's open sliding door, clumsily shielding our purchases under our jackets.

I crawled inside, over Adelaide's car seat, which I had not yet allowed anyone to remove, and was mildly surprised to find my brother-in-law, Marky, in the driver's seat, and Miguel in the far back, his face slack and emotionless.

"What's going on? Are you okay?" A stupid question considering our daughter had only died three days earlier—but even so, this was unusual behavior for Miguel.

"Uh, Jeffrey and Tommy just called to offer me Broadway."

"Wait, what? But I thought . . ." My voice got lost in my thoughts as the rippling effects of this news settled over me. I adopted Miguel's dazed expression as I crawled between the car seats and into the way back to join him.

Shock, table for two?

Jeffrey, aka Jeffrey Seller, the lead producer on *Hamilton,* and Tommy, aka Thomas Kail, the Tony Award–winning director of the original *Hamilton* production, had made the offer personally. This was an honor; it was also a lifeline. Several months earlier, it had been announced that *Hamilton* in Chicago would close on January 5, 2020, and we had absolutely no idea what we were going to do for money on January 6th. We weren't concerned in the short term, as we had money saved and this was the natural ebb and flow of the theater business that we reluctantly accepted. Though in the past, we had always had my career to fall back on.

"Everything okay?" My mother asked, turning around in the front passenger seat.

"Um, I was just offered Hamilton on Broadway," Miguel answered, still dazed.

"Oh . . . wow." Like a contagion, our overwhelmed and uncertain expressions spread to my mom's face. I couldn't see Marky's face as he stayed focused on the road in front of him, but I imagined he had also been infected.

Under any other circumstance, what we were going to do post-*Hamilton* in Chicago would have been the most pressing conversation in our lives: Do we stay in Chicago where all of Adelaide's doctors are? But how do we make a living? Do we move back to NYC where Miguel has a better chance of booking another job? But what would that mean for Adelaide's care? However, given Adelaide's declining health when the closing date was announced, we'd barely addressed the topic. We had been surviving each day; the future felt abstract and, if not irrelevant, at least insignificant.

The offer to continue to play Hamilton on Broadway was great news, amazing news even: we now had stability, security, and a logical path forward. But in that moment, all we saw was the monumental change awaiting us, and we were already at capacity for processing major life changes.

"Couldn't they have waited to call until after her service at least?" I asked.

"The guy playing Hamilton *just* put in his notice to leave this morning. I imagine they thought we could use some good news."

We both knew there was no way we could say no to this opportunity, but I couldn't imagine leaving Chicago, where Adelaide had spent a majority of her life, where we had built a community that we loved and who loved us in return. A community that knew Adelaide in ways no one else ever would and had supported us through the wildest years I hope I ever experience. How would we leave this life behind and not feel like we were leaving Adelaide with it? How would I reconcile so much loss in such close proximity to such a windfall of fortune?

I quickly decided these were future Kelly's problems and resisted talking about the job offer and the impending move for as long as possible. Despite my hovering around in the denial stage, over the next few weeks a plan formed: we would ease back into East Coast life with Miguel returning in March 2020 to perform on Broadway, taking turns going back and forth between our new home in Jersey and our condo in Chicago until the end of the summer, when Jackson and I would join Miguel permanently in time for the new school year.

While becoming a single parent for six months while still in the darkest days of my grief was not super high on my bucket list, it would allow Jackson to finish out school with his friends and me to drag out moving away from Chicago for as long as possible (bargaining stage, anyone?). That is, until we started hearing news reports about a contagious virus spreading out of Wuhan, China. Miguel got in ten performances on Broadway before the world shut down and he returned to us in Chicago, where we quarantined for the next four months.

Ah, those early days when we thought the kids would be back in school in two weeks and that Miguel would be back on stage even sooner. Alas, two mortgage payments and no foreseeable income does not a happy bank account make, and by early summer we decided to sell our Chicago condo earlier than anticipated and begin preparing to move back to New Jersey. All in the middle of an unprecedented global pandemic. There would be nothing gradual about moving back. Instead, the Band-Aid would be ripped off in one swift and searing motion.

Bracing for the pain, I put my head down and bulldozed forward, not allowing myself to ruminate on what was happening. To a large extent it was out of my control, anyway. Adelaide's room needed to be packed up, so I packed it. Her medications that had remained untouched in a kitchen cabinet for the last eight months needed to be sorted, so I sorted them. There wasn't time, or I didn't make time, to process how returning to New Jersey would emotionally affect me (*aaand* we're back to denial). I decided that the feelings would come and I just needed to ride the wave. In theory this was smart, as anticipating grief doesn't lessen or amplify the experience of it. However, because I hadn't given it much thought, I was completely unprepared for the tsunami that hit me on Interstate 78 as our car, containing all our earthly possessions that were not currently packed on a moving truck, drove closer and closer to our New Jersey home.

It was 10 PM, we had twenty more minutes to go, and I was driving the last leg. Miguel was scrolling on his phone beside me and, thankfully, Jackson was passed out behind us, so he didn't witness what was, perhaps, inevitable. As each exit flew by, my brain began spiraling faster and faster: here we were, our little family returning to New Jersey after nearly four years away—but we had left as a family of four and were returning as (at least physically) a family of three.

In the rearview mirror I looked at where Adelaide's car seat had been. Where she should have been. We had Adelaide cremated since I didn't want to bury her in Chicago when I knew we would be moving. So, in our car, in her little box, she came with us—but this was not how it was supposed to be.

As the surroundings began to look more and more familiar, my chest tightened. I gripped the wheel in an attempt to stop my shaking hands. And then my peripheral vision began to blur.

"Mig, I need you to drive now." I felt him looking at me, registering my physical and emotional changes in real time.

"Okay, you're going to be okay, just find a place to pull over."

Not able to wait for an exit ramp, I flicked on the hazards and guided our car onto the interstate shoulder. When I was finally in the safety of the passenger seat, I let go of the many strings I had been trying to hold together inside my head and chest while operating the four thousand pounds of metal containing everything I hold dear. What escaped my body was not traditional waterworks, but explosive hyperventilating sobs.

"Please, Miguel, I can't do this," I pleaded in between gasping breaths. "Let's go back. I want to go back home. I want to go home. I want to go home. I want to go home."

My chest felt like it might implode. I was shaking uncontrollably. I couldn't breathe, I couldn't see—*I couldn't do this*. I couldn't move back without my daughter. I couldn't reunite with old friends who hadn't held her and experienced her nuzzling in closer, or connected with her on a rare moment when she had opened her eyes. I couldn't meet new people who would never know her.

"We can't go back. We have to go forward. We're almost ho—at the new house," Miguel caught himself. "It's going to be okay. You're going to be okay. Just try to breathe." Then he looked in the rearview mirror to be sure that Jackson was still asleep, and I felt the sharp sting of shame.

What would Jackson think if he had witnessed this? How would it affect him to see his mother so out of control? What kind of mother was I? I knew we weren't going back to Chicago. I knew I wasn't just Adelaide's mother, that Jackson needed me too. I knew we had a new home now.

Fifteen minutes later, and after spiraling through shock, denial, anger, and bargaining, we were pulling into our New Jersey driveway. I finally regained control of my breathing, grateful that a groggy Jackson had been spared from what could have been a traumatizing scene. I stayed in the acceptance stage just long enough to unpack the car. This transition was going to be really freaking hard, and in a move of utter surrender, I rarely left my bed over the next few days. (Hello depression stage, my old friend.)

When I zoom in on this one major life change experienced amidst the throes of grief, I can see Kübler-Ross's model at work. With the model in mind, I can see how I might better prepare for challenging transitions in the future— perhaps by doing a little processing *before* I get in the car to move away from nearly every memory of my daughter.

Whether change is thrust upon you or is patiently waiting until you're ready, it has to happen eventually. You can face it and move forward, backward, and diagonally through it, and come out on the other side—or maybe you are hedging your bets that you will never be forced to empty that closet or go through those drawers. You figure that you have endured enough change, and the rest of life can stay just the way it is. But you don't need me to remind you how unhealthy that is. It is never the well-adjusted and happy character in the movie that has the untouched time capsule of a room hidden behind the locked door.

So, what if, instead of using the word "change," which has all sorts of negatively charged emotions attached to it, we swap it out for "evolve" or "adapt"? We are taught in school about evolution and "survival of the fittest," and our society often considers the "fittest" to be the strongest, smartest, or healthiest—but that is not what Charles Darwin meant. As Leon Megginson paraphrases, survival of the fittest means that "it is not the most intellectual of the species that survives; it is not the strongest that survives; but the species that survives is the one that is able best to **adapt** and adjust to the changing environment in which it finds itself." And Darwin's theory of natural selection, as defined by the *Oxford Advanced Learner's Dictionary*, is "the process by which plants, animals, etc., that can **adapt** to their environment survive and produce young, while the others disappear [emphasis added]."

Tyrannosaurus rex, one of the strongest and most ferocious animals to roam the earth, died out. There were a number of other human species inhabiting the earth 300,000 years ago with intelligence likely comparable to *Homo sapiens*.[12] However, *Homo sapiens* survived, becoming modern humans, and the rest did not.

You know what did survive?

Cockroaches.

Cockroaches survived the asteroid that destroyed the dinosaurs, they survived multiple ice ages, and they are even surviving human-caused environmental changes. A study out of North Carolina State University found that not only are cockroaches able to adjust their internal chemistry to survive, but they can do it in just a few generations.[13] New environment, new aggressor, lack of traditional food source? No problem, cockroaches will have modified their DNA in time for their grandchildren to thrive. Look, I get it, cockroaches aren't exactly sexy, and I'm pretty sure few people have ever taken being called a cockroach as a compliment. But when it comes to surviving change, it absolutely should be.

Which brings me back to Kübler-Ross's final stages: acceptance and processing. In order to effectively navigate our grief, we must *accept* the change that has occurred in our life. Then we have to channel our inner cockroach and *process* the change in order to survive it. Similar to the evolution of cockroaches, it may feel like we are being changed on a cellular level. I know you know this, but it bears repeating here: you cannot go back to who you were. You can only go forward as who you are now. It is that new and adapted person that will survive.

Change forces us to adapt. Packing away their belongings forces us to adapt to our loved one's minimized physical presence in our lives. Moving holiday celebrations to a new home when the person who usually hosts is no longer with us forces us to adapt to new traditions. None of this is easy, and we don't have to like that our person takes up less space in our lives—but we do have to accept that it is our new reality. Though I have to admit it hasn't stopped me from feeling Adelaide and remembering her in every room of our new home. I don't need to keep all her hair bows in a drawer to remember braiding her hair on our couch in Chicago. I don't have to hold on to her therapy toys to remember the joy I felt when she finally pushed the button releasing the little blue elephant from its chamber all on her own.

One of the final pieces of wisdom I take from Kübler-Ross is less about recognizing which phase I'm currently in and more about how grieving is a universal experience. At any given point, someone who is mourning will be negotiating one of the seven stages, even if they are unsure which one or are unaware that the stages even exist. There is something comforting in the normalcy of grief. In knowing that, as difficult as it is to lose someone and face the resulting changes to and in our lives, our emotions, resistance, and the ensuing journey are all part of the process. Change is constant, and eventually we must adjust and adapt to our new present no matter how much we dislike it. After all, it is not the strongest or the smartest among us that will thrive—it is the motherfucking cockroaches.

How do you feel about the Kübler-Ross stages? Do they help you to articulate or better understand your grief? What about your feelings around change? Are there certain changes closely associated with your grief that have been particularly messy?

Writing about my I-78 panic attack as if it were a scene in a novel helped to put some distance between me and the experience so that I could better understand what I was feeling through the lens of the grief stages. If helpful, try writing about your situation as if you were in a novel or screenplay.

If these prompts don't connect with you, feel free to write about anything that does.

7

When Your Greatest Fear Is Socializing

What do you say? There really are no words for that. There really aren't. Somebody tries to say, "I'm sorry, I'm so sorry." People say that to me. There's no language for it. Sorry doesn't do it. I think you should just hug people and mop their floor or something.

—Toni Morrison

There's a general impulse to distract the grieving person—as if you could.

—Joan Didion

There will inevitably be questions and conversations that elicit the worst of our grief. *Are you married? Do your parents live nearby? What are you doing for the holidays? How many children do you have?* Anticipating having to answer these questions can be socially crippling. I found myself wishing I lived two hundred years ago when people still wore all black as a sign of mourning. Not for nothing did past societies have a much healthier relationship with death and loss than we do today. Of course, they were confronted with death more frequently thanks to a lack of medical knowledge and poor hygiene—but there is still something to be learned from that time and how plainly they communicated about death and grief.

Given that we were not living in the 1800s, my first line of defense in avoiding any grief-provoking questions was to send Miguel out as our strong, first-string lineman to meet everyone and tell them about our shrunken family so that I didn't have to. I knew this was unfair to Miguel and also only a short-term solution—that, eventually, I would have to answer questions about our family on my own. But at the time this was the best I could come up with.

Language around death is challenging enough as it is. Do I have to use "was" instead of "is"? What happens if I trip up? What if I just don't feel like referring to Adelaide in the past tense? And this is all swimming around in my head before I even utter a word to someone in public. I quickly discovered that there are no verb tense police who are going to ticket me for using the incorrect tense, so if I feel like saying Adelaide "is" one day, and "was" the next, then I can do whatever I damn well please.

If only the other aspects of communicating about death were as straightforward.

I'm convinced that there are two types of people in this world: the people that rehearse difficult conversations in the car, or the shower, or in front of their bathroom mirror, and the people who wing them. I have always been the former and, prior to Bluetooth connections in cars, definitely got a few off looks from neighboring drivers as they caught me playing out deeply dramatic interactions with invisible boyfriends or frenemies while waiting for a light to change. The exchange in real life, if it ever even happened, rarely played out the way I had rehearsed, but I absolutely felt more confident walking into it.

So, as the weeks rolled by, I did what any former performer-type would do: I rehearsed. I practiced all sorts of scenarios where Adelaide might come up when meeting someone new and the different ways I could respond. Miguel reminded me that I always had the option to say that I had one child and not mention Adelaide at all. He said that he would gauge the situation as it was unfolding and decide whether it was something that he wanted to get into with that person or if it was easier to let it slide by unsaid.

I understood this tactic and even appreciated it. But no matter how deeply I thought I wanted to avoid these conversations about the death of my child, there was no way I could bring myself to deny her existence even through omission—nor did I want to.

"Why, Kelly? Why do you have to bring her up if it's only going to hurt you to talk about her?" Miguel asked.

It took a while to find the reason, but when I did, my stubbornness on the issue made more sense: "Because I want everyone to know about Adelaide. To know she existed. To know that she is a part of our family even if they will never meet her. To understand that she is a part of us and, even in her absence, defines who we are."

"Sure, but even if it's just small talk?"

"Yep, even then."

As discussed in chapter four, we all grieve differently. So, for some people, Miguel's tactic of determining how much to share in the moment makes sense. They know the truth—that their loved one was here and existed. They don't need social acquaintances to verify or acknowledge that for them.

It must be nice to be so secure. I wouldn't know. So, I rehearsed.

But then there were the times that the anticipation of The Conversation was so heavy and ominous that I would prompt the discussion by asking the other person how many children they had. This way I wouldn't feel sucker punched when the difficult questions arose. I was inviting them, addressing them, and moving forward with my truth in the open. Once I realized how much control I had over these conversations, they became less anxiety-inducing and draining. Because the truth of the matter was that I wanted to talk about Adelaide—after all, it was the other person's loss that they never got to know her. Also, if I wanted to change the topic, I could.

We instinctively know the questions, comments, and scenarios that amplify our grief until it feels like we've swallowed a baseball. As with so many aspects of our grief, the suspense while waiting for difficult moments can be so much worse than the moments themselves. If that's true for you, instead of preemptively obsessing over them, why not prepare for them? Put into words what fears or concerns are making your heart race, and then find ways to either work around them or address them head-on. Knowing exactly how you are going to respond in these situations, be it at the office, playground, or grocery store, will help build your confidence—or at the very least, shrink that baseball down to a nice manageable golf ball.

The conversations will probably still be awkward, the anxiety still present, but we have the power to control these conversations. With a little preparation and repetitive practice, they do not have to slay us.

My initial social anxiety had been sparked by meeting new people and having to find the words to explain Adelaide and her loss. But now that I had my script ready to go, I should have felt more confident, right? Ha! This time, though, the anxiety source was less obvious and would take me months to figure out.

As time moved forward without my permission, further distancing me from life with my daughter, I noticed a growing desire to talk about her. It would start as a simple thought of her in conversation, something that reminded of me of her—six degrees of Adelaide Grace, though it rarely took that many. But what began as an itch developed into an urgent burn the longer the conversation went on. I fought against it, in part because I didn't want to be *that* person who obsessively talks about their loss. The Debbie Downer that people pitied, were sometimes annoyed by, and most of the time avoided.

But I *was* obsessed. I was desperate to talk about her, to remember her and make sure everyone I came into contact with remembered her as well. Time was rushing past me, and the separation between then and now was growing alarmingly wide. As if I stood on one peak staring across a valley to the opposing peak of my former life. The only thing connecting the two was a taut rope that lengthened with each passing day. However, I noticed that the more I spoke about her, the slower the rope grew, and I hoped that maybe I could pull the two peaks closer together or, at a minimum, prevent them from growing farther apart.

It was more than that, though. I didn't just want them to know that she had died; I needed them to know that she had lived. That she was more than a devastating chapter in my life story, that she was vibrant and engaging and that she left an impression on all who met her. Was talking about her the healing salve I was craving? In some ways it was—the itch would be soothed for a short while. The price was steep, though, and paid in the currency of sheer anxiety.

Why, though? Why did speaking about someone I loved, someone I *wanted* to talk about, drive up my heart rate?

I didn't have the answers—but my eight-year-old did.

"That movie looks scary!"

Jackson and I were negotiating a movie selection. A year into the pandemic, we were running low on family-friendly entertainment that could captivate us both. I swear, the ultimate test for any international negotiator should be arbitrating a family movie night.

"You have watched far scarier movies, and besides, you know those monsters aren't real." Nothing like peer pressure from your mother.

"It's not the monsters I'm scared of, it's the people's reactions to them."

I stared back, dumbfounded. Well, shit.

Once I got over the fact that my son is clearly an emotional sage, I applied his acute understanding of his fear to my own. I could memorize a rehearsed monologue in preparation for emotionally fraught questions or conversations; I could even long for them to occur and offer an excuse to share my daughter's memory with the world—but I couldn't prepare myself for how people would respond.

My grief might as well have been some lurking sea monster and I its inevitable first victim. For me, my grief was familiar, a known factor. Did it try to eat me alive sometimes? Sure, but somehow I always survived. The mystery— the fear—lay in how others responded.

I didn't even need to wait for their responses. Anticipating them was more than enough. Would they say something upsetting to me? Would they feel unnecessarily guilty for bringing her up? Would tears cloud their eyes and I would end up consoling *them* or brushing off *their* concern? At some point, anticipating the responses to my grief had become far more anxiety-inducing than talking about the reason for my grief itself.

It's not the monsters I'm scared of, it's the people's reactions to them.

Our society places so much weight on trying to fix or resolve issues when they are brought to us. Everyone has their own expert advice—look no further than all the political, pandemic, and international affairs armchair aficionados roaming Twitter. They read one exposé in the *Guardian* and are instantly experts. It is no wonder that this inherent need to fix and advise would translate into our personal lives as well. I became proficient at navigating these conversations during my daughter's life:

"Yes, we have tried CBD."

"No, I don't think your sister's essential oil business could help her."

"I'm so sorry to hear about your dog's seizures, but my daughter is a human, so . . ."

The reality is that there are certain situations where little can be said in one conversation, post, tweet, or comment that is going to relieve someone's pain or struggle. Especially when it comes to grief. And that's assuming the hurting person is even looking to be healed.

Until someone has experienced deep grief directly, it is hard for them to understand that instead of trying to fix the situation (which is impossible), it is often best to just acknowledge how crappy it is. But, unfortunately, this isn't typically how these conversations go. So it's up to the griever to prepare . . . again.

"God only gives us what we can handle."

"They're in a better place now."

"Heaven needed another angel."

Sentiments like these, among others, devalue the legitimate pain that someone is feeling. They can come across like someone is making an excuse for the death of our loved ones. Making it smaller or brushing it off because it was meant to be.

Sentiments like these are also *not true*.

I *couldn't* handle my sick daughter, which was why I advocated for home nursing and why, since her passing, I am in therapy and on anti-depressants. As for heaven's needs? I have a decidedly difficult time believing that, after billions and billions of lives lived and lost, heaven is struggling with occupancy rates.

As I am processing their words and debating my response, a palpable anger floods my systems—how could someone presume that they had the power to tidy up such a catastrophic loss with some pat trope? As if (a) I had never heard that before; or (b) this time, coming from them, it would make it all okay. This is chased by a torrent of guilt because the person's intent was to comfort me, right? They are just trying to help me in the best way they know how.

But were they really?

Hear me out.

The more I pushed through these interactions and all their conflicting emotions, the more I realized that often the person's intention was not necessarily to make me feel better, but to relieve themselves of their own sadness and guilt. So, I started referring to these types of conversations as intention conventions. Before I would let myself get upset by the other person's use of simple, yet harmful, sayings, I would ask myself what the person's intention was. It was almost never to hurt me; in fact, if they knew that was exactly what they had done, they would probably be devastated. No, their intention was to offer condolences—albeit shallow ones—and to make my grief go away so that it would make them less uncomfortable.

Once I was able to recognize that these unhelpful and tired responses had little to do with me and everything to do with them, I worked on not letting their efforts (or lack thereof) affect me. I thanked them and moved on, leaving their emotional baggage where it belonged: with them. Goodness knows my load is heavy enough as it is.

Then there were the people who would feel guilty for bringing Adelaide up or start crying at the impact of such a loss. What was their intention? Again, their response wasn't about me—it was about how it affected them. It was a sign of their uncomfortableness with loss and grief, or perhaps it pinched the nerve of their greatest fears.

At first, I felt a need to comfort this other person, as if their emotional response was somehow my fault. "It's okay, she had a rough life. We're doing better now." But that felt dishonest, because what happened to her wasn't okay, and neither was I. Also, why was I brushing off this life-altering loss? That was *exactly* what I despised about the well-meaning but overused sayings I'd heard too many times before.

Other times I would hug them, but, wow, that was super awkward. *Here, let me comfort you about my dead daughter* . . . hard pass.

Yes, their response was attached to their own personal lived experiences, but just as I wanted my loss to be witnessed and acknowledged, I found witnessing their response helped make me feel a little less like the grief Godzilla chasing down innocent civilians.

"Oh my gosh, I'm so, so sorry." Their eyes become glassy, as if on cue.

I'd say, "Thank you. It really sucked. Still sucks, honestly. But we're working through it. She was an amazing little lady. So fierce and feisty. You should have seen her swat at her brother when she was sick of him cuddling her."

Then, if the person's emotional baggage was too much, they could change the subject. If not, then I had opened the door for us to talk about her, which was what I truly wanted.

In time, I also found validation in these strong emotional responses. Yes, their tears were awkward, but in all the ways that someone saying "At least she's in a better place" felt dismissive (*perhaps she is, Dave, but I'm not!*), their tears showed me they understood the gravity of my loss. Not that I want to be regularly comforting strangers during get-to-know-you conversations, but I can find comfort, or something in that vein, by acknowledging that they see me.

While conversing with strangers about grief can be upsetting and disappointing, it doesn't compare to the disappointment that we feel when talking with friends who can't seem to get it, or, more likely, don't want to.

We all have a certain tolerance level for the uncomfortable. Like anything in life, the more we endure, the higher our tolerance level rises. So, it makes sense that those who have endured a significant loss would have a much higher tolerance for another person's uncomfortable grief. But it can be shocking when someone who you thought was a BFF is now MIA. It may start with them trying to diminish your grief or avoiding the topic altogether. Maybe they stop answering your calls, or because they are not an empathetic, present, or patient support, you stop calling them and naturally, over time, the distance grows. Other times the split can be far more dramatic and include arguments or blunt rejection. As with grief, the more this friend, or, heaven forbid, family member, means to us, the more the loss of their love and support hurts. It also just sucks that now, on top of your loved one dying, you are also grieving a friendship. It's bullshit, really.

(I was fortunate, in a backhanded sort of way, that I weeded through my contact list when Adelaide was diagnosed. It also helped that not long after her diagnosis we moved halfway across the country, so all the new people in our life met us with Adelaide as she was. If you couldn't take my family at our frequent hospitalizations and seizures, then you didn't get us at our *Hamilton*, exciting events, and cute family photos. By the time Adelaide died, I knew that the people who had stuck around were lifers.)

As devastating as these additional losses can be, especially when we are already at our lowest, I have found it best to just let the person go. Grieve the relationship, try to find some sort of peace with it, and then move forward. It is excruciating, upsetting, and unbelievably frustrating, but you can't make someone be something they aren't. How lucky they are that they have not yet had to build up their tolerance for the uncomfortable. Someday they will, though, and hopefully they will have people around them who have a higher tolerance than they once did. Until then, you can send them a Grief Awareness Day greeting card every August 30th.

It all comes down to remembering that we cannot control how someone will respond to learning about our grief. Nor can we let an anticipated response prevent us from sharing our loved ones' memory with the world. (Though maybe I can filter some of those memories into a journal or call a friend or loved one who gets it so that I don't become a word-vomiting King Kong clinging to the peak on the other side of that vast valley.)

I can control how I let the responses affect me. I can let well-intentioned but ignorant comments roll off my back—they are not about me. I can let people know that I actually enjoy talking about my child, regardless of whether she's still physically with me—after all, what parent doesn't love an excuse to gush about their children?—and that her memory has just as much joy attached to it as pain. Or, I can even change the subject and walk away. There are so many options that *are* within my control. Recognizing this has been empowering enough to ease anxiety's viselike grip on my social interactions.

My grief may look like an invincible monster in need of vanquishing, but it's really just another form of that rope tethering me to my mountain of memories. To the joy, hope, sadness, and anger of a lost love. We don't need to be afraid of our monsters . . . or the people who meet them.

You're talking with someone new, and *that* question comes up. What is the question for you?

Let's say you answer it honestly. What is the response you wish to hear? What is the response you fear most? How do you let each response affect your day?

If these prompts don't connect with you, feel free to write about anything that does.

8

When You Feel Alone

Deep grief sometimes is almost like a specific location, a coordinate on a map of time. When you are standing in that forest of sorrow, you cannot imagine that you could ever find your way to a better place. But if someone can assure you that they themselves have stood in that same place, and now have moved on, sometimes this will bring hope.

—Elizabeth Gilbert

We bereaved are not alone. We belong to the largest company in all the world—the company of those who have known suffering.

—Helen Keller

You somehow find the energy and courage to leave your home and are met by a world that continues to go on while your personal corner of it feels frozen in time. Friends and family may try to understand, but unless they've experienced a similar loss, how could they? And even people who could be in a different stage of their grief or are grieving their loss differently from you. Grief can be an intrinsically isolating experience: it is draining, depressing, and makes you feel undesirable. The lack of control we have over when it surfaces can make us feel like a werewolf under a full moon. Yet, despite—or because of—how isolating it can feel, we are often desperate to share our grief with someone, anyone, who will understand.

Friends of ours were having a small, COVID-compliant birthday party for their daughter, who was turning three—and, since Adelaide had been three when she died, I knew this could potentially be difficult for me. I had already learned that, whenever I attended any gathering at any event or venue outside my home, I needed to take stock of the bathrooms or quiet corners where I could escape should I feel my inner werewolf coming out. But thanks to COVID, this party was outside, leaving me with little space for private lycanthropy.

Before we arrived, I explained to Miguel that, when we were at the party and I told him it was time to go, he needed to listen and *leave*—not linger with long goodbyes as he was wont to do. We were among good friends, friends who knew Adelaide, who loved us and supported us. This was a safe environment. But still, I wasn't eager to go gushing my grief all over their daughter's special day. Through most of the party I held it together and was so freaking proud of myself—until it was time to sing happy birthday.

"Happy birthday to me! I'm free!!!" their daughter sang out.

It happened quickly, a new crack opening in my heart, pressure building from within. I looked at Miguel across the patio and nodded toward the fence gate. He said our goodbyes while I gathered our things. We stepped out of their yard and I focused on our car across the street. I just needed to make it to our car: one step, another step, one step more. Once we were inside our car, my tears pooled. I couldn't stop them anymore, but I tried to keep them silent. As we drove past their house, Miguel rolled down the window to wave one last goodbye, unaware that I was losing it beside him. I hid my face behind Miguel's body and waved my arm, the lone limb that hadn't fully werewolfed, enthusiastically.

My chest was tight, a howl building within. This grief was painful, my heart breaking in real time. I needed to explode, but I didn't want to do that in front of Jackson. I had to hold it together just a little bit longer, so I dug my fingernails into my thigh trying to focus on the physical pain instead of the emotional. It was working. I released my leg and saw the indentions my nails left in my thigh, like a real-life werewolf making its mark. Miguel looked over at me and I can only imagine the disaster he saw in front of him: the werewolf desperately holding on to her humanity. He squeezed my left hand as I dug the nails on my right back into my thigh.

We pulled into our driveway and, as soon as the car rolled to a stop, I was out of its steel confines and running inside. Miguel called after me asking if I was okay.

No, I'm not okay! I'm a freaking werewolf!

I kicked my shoes off and ran upstairs to my office, which was adorned with items from Adelaide's room in Chicago. With the door closed, my howling sobs erupted. I tried to deafen them with a pillow, sucking in air through the fibers of the pillowcase. It was hard to breathe, but I didn't care. I needed to get the pain out of my chest. Without the pillow, Jackson would have heard. It might have scared him—he would have wanted to help me, but nothing could help me. I just needed to get the pain out. It didn't last long—a few minutes—then I lay there, staring out the window. I turned on the audio recording of Adelaide's oxygen concentrator (because grief is weird) and allowed myself to be comforted by the familiar whooshing sounds while gazing at the tree branches outside the window. They weren't moving—not a single leaf was even ruffled. For once, time in the outside world seemed to match time inside my cocoon.

Looking back at the party, no one made me feel like I didn't fit in, like I was different. I had been in the company of close friends who knew of my pain even if they couldn't understand it, and still I felt lonely, out of place, and like I needed to run away. In fact, I didn't just feel like I had to run away—I literally had.

I had run to the safety of a private space before my werewolf took over, and I'd made it—but it had been a close call. We can't always make it to a safe space, away from innocent onlookers, before our fangs grow and claws sharpen. What then? There isn't much we can do at that point except ride it out and hope we don't do too much damage in the interim. What I will say is that most of the public werewolfing stories I have heard end in the comforting arms of a stranger. Probably not ideal, but perhaps unexpectedly comforting. The human experience is no stranger to grief—even in a small group of people there will be at least one who understands. One who is also a secret werewolf, one who will sit with you until it passes. Even at peak were-ferocity, we are still human.

Still, I wanted to limit potential public breakdowns, so following my lycanthropic near miss, I knew I needed to try something new to tame my inner grief beast. I just wasn't sure what.

"Hi Kelly, looking forward to having you at our November retreat . . ."

Retreat? In a cinematic flood of images, I saw the previous night's activities roll out before me: glasses of wine, the social media doomscrolling, the message from a relative stranger suggesting this particular grief retreat for mothers who'd lost a child—which just so happened to be an accessible two-hour drive from our home *and* happened to have just one last spot available for their November session—which was less than two months away.

Oh God, what had I done?

I'll tell you what I had never done before: participate in group therapy or anything resembling the like. The closest I had come to what I thought of as forced group bonding had been when I pledged a sorority in my freshman year of college. I dropped out before initiation, which had led to a candlelit ambush by my pledge sisters pleading for me to stay. So, not a great track record . . . and it forever tainted Cyndi Lauper's "True Colors" for me.

"I think it will be good for you," my mother said.

I just figured that if it was awful it would at least give me some solid writing material.

So, a few weeks later, I pulled up to a gorgeous house in the middle of nowhere, New Jersey, and reminded myself that none of these women knew each other either and were also scared and hurting. (Still, was it too late to turn around and go home?)

I gathered my overnight bag and my courage and walked in the open front door. There were a few women gathered in the kitchen chatting and laughing, but I was stopped, before I reached them, by one of the retreat directors who pointed me upstairs in the direction of my room where I could drop my bag.

"You have two other roommates; I think you'll really like them."

The room was large and well-lit, with four twin beds and an en suite bathroom. One of the beds had a bag on it, and on the nightstand next to it sat a framed picture of a teenage girl who I could tell had various disabilities. A daughter, I knew, who was no longer with her mother.

I had been so focused on my own grief, I hadn't thought much about what losses had brought the other ten women here. Or that this weekend would also be about holding space for their grief, their guilt, and the finer points in between. Anxiety entered my heart, as if injected by a syringe, and I immediately questioned my mother's advice to attend. (Since certainly *someone* was to blame for my current predicament.) Was carrying the intimate details of ten other mothers' stories really good for me?

"Get settled and then we'll meet in the living room in ten minutes, ladies!" A voice called from the bottom of the stairs.

Deep breath.

No turning back now . . . I guess.

I put my bag on one of the free beds and took out my own framed photo: Adelaide in the light green dress she was going to wear as the flower girl in our friends' wedding, but instead wore to her impromptu fourth birthday party the week before she passed.

I stared at the photo while I willed my heart rate to slow. *Oh, my sweet girl, what have you gotten me into?*

However, despite all my trepidations, the weekend was far from awful. Emotional, tragic, gut-wrenching? For sure. But it was also beautiful, cleansing, and, dare I say it, healing.

Over the course of the next two days, we shared about our families; our child(ren) we'd lost and how we lost them; how it affected our relationships, our lives, our remaining children, and loved ones. We did campy art projects and basic yoga together, dined at a communal table, and slept three or four to a room. There was nothing out of the ordinary or disturbing, no chanting or indoctrination—just talking and bonding. At any given point there was usually someone crying, and no one wondered why. They would simply offer a tissue and a hug, question- and judgment-free.

We came to that house from a variety of cultural, financial, political, and religious backgrounds. We ranged in ages over two decades and came from as far away as South Dakota. The only thing we all had in common was that we had all lost a child—but even then, how old our child had been and what had taken them varied from mother to mother. Nonetheless, our enduring experience was strong enough to bind us together.

Our second and final night, we huddled under blankets around a firepit on the back deck of the house. The moon's light reflected ethereally off both the lake bordering the backyard and our alcohol. One of the retreat leaders (who, like all of the leaders, had also lost a child) brought a music speaker to our now boisterous conversation and proceeded to curate a playlist mostly consisting of '90s hip-hop and bubblegum pop. We danced, sang, lip-synced, and Tootsee Rolled the night away. For a few hours, we were free of our grief and guilt, letting go in a way many of us hadn't been able to do in years. Under the light of that moon, we were no longer lone werewolves. We had found our pack.

With everyone else in my life, and most definitely with new people I met, I felt like I had been broken and put back together to form a person who no longer fit in with regular, non-grieving people. But with these women, these equally broken mothers, I was *normal* broken. They didn't see me as a pariah made of grief. They expected nothing more from me than what I was capable of giving in that moment, nor I of them. And if I suddenly burst into tears, someone would come to hold my hand while the conversation continued. Here our grief was welcomed. Here we were all normal broken together.

These women also reminded me of one of my guiding truths: I am just not that special. Is there someone out there that found out her daughter had epilepsy the same week her husband booked the role of Hamilton, moved across the country for said role, fought tooth and nail for her daughter, lost her to an unknown neurodegenerative condition three years later, then found out she had to move back across the country because her husband was going to be Hamilton on Broadway? Probably not. That story is uniquely mine.

But have other people fought for their medically complex child? Have other people lost a child or a loved one? Have others had to move cross-country several times for a spouse's job while abandoning their own dreams? Absolutely. I am still unique in all the ways Mr. Rogers taught me, but I'm not under any misconception that I am special enough to be the only person feeling the way I do. My grief, my anger, my determination, my joy, and all the thoughts that come along with them are not unique to me. I am not brave in sharing them because I know I am not alone in feeling them. I am just not *that* special.

It is this realization that led me to share our family's story publicly on network news and privately on phone calls, where I could validate the thoughts and frustrations of families with newly diagnosed children. It is what allowed me to connect with the other mothers at the retreat and what motivated me to write this book. There is nothing on these pages that someone else hasn't also felt before. How liberating is that? We are not terrible humans for feeling any of the multitude of supposedly negative emotions or having any of the impulsive, drastic, or depressing thoughts that cross our minds. We are human and we are not alone. Only by expressing these emotions to people who understand can we relinquish their hold on us.

Okay, so, there are people out there that can relate to you and you to them. The tricky part can be finding them. And as awkward and deflating as social media can be, it is a great place to start. Search through hashtags of loss categorically similar to yours, start following people who are on a similar grief journey, comment on their posts, introduce yourself in DMs.

If you prefer to live IRL, Google a grief retreat. There are so many amazing ones out there that will directly connect you with people who are normal broken, just like you, for one long, terrifying, and inescapable weekend. Many offer scholarships so that they are free to attend outside of travel costs. Hospitals often have grief groups too, and even if you decide that the whole group thing isn't for you, maybe there is one person at one session that you can connect with outside of the group.

Also, take note when your friend says that they have a friend that went through something similar and take them up on an introduction. Will it be awkward at first? Possibly. But the more people you know who are on a similar journey, the less lonely you will feel. It is these people who get it, who will listen to you or will sit in silence with you. Your tears won't scare them away, nor will they try to rush you through them. They won't try to fix you, but instead they will accept you as you are.

These friendships are the most effective when they can be reciprocated. There is a special kind of healing that takes place when you can sit with someone else in their dark place and be their werewolf remedy. In fact, this healing-through-helping salve has been well studied and documented. A 2006 study conducted by Jorge Moll and Frank Krueger found that giving money, goods, or time activates a part of the brain that also happens to get excited about food and sex.[14] Gives new meaning to the phrase "giving feels good," no?

By helping us feel better for just a moment, helping others gives us enough of a break in the clouds to push forward on our healing journey. Through the sun's rays, hope seeps into our skin like a vitamin as we are given the opportunity to grow something positive out of our tragedy. To create meaning and give us a reason to get out of bed in the morning. It's no wonder that many nonprofits are started in memory of someone who has been lost. But our acts of kindness don't need to be as grand as filing for our own 501(c)(3); it could be volunteering for a cause that is near to our hearts, bringing a coworker an unexpected cup of coffee, or being that judgment-free ear or shoulder for someone else who is grieving.

Maybe it's because of those food and sex activators, or maybe it's because we are nurturing positivity where destruction and despair once reigned, but we are creating purpose from pain. Be it a grand world-saving endeavor or a simpler day-brightening effort—helping is healing.

To be clear, the loss of our loved one will never be worth it. I have met so many incredible individuals and families over the course of Adelaide's illness and death. The good Adelaide inspired me to do in the world, the people I have helped, the fact that this book even exists—that's all because I knew and loved her. None of this, nor the happiness and purpose I've pulled from it, would exist if she hadn't suffered and been lost. And yet I would give it all up to have her back with me healthy and happy.

Still, I continue trying to connect with others and to turn something super shitty into a moment of hope for someone else and, in turn, an ounce of healing for me.

Whether we are clinging to our normal broken community or they are leaning on us, these reciprocal relationships help us understand our grief and feel a little less alone in a world that is seemingly moving on without us. Simply knowing that my normal broken people are out there is enough for me to prevent future unexpected werewolf transformations. It's not just that I need them, it's that I know they need me too. Of course, every now and then, the beast will take over—and that's natural. But it no longer causes me anxiety wondering when and where it will happen. I can interact with friends who are fortunate enough to not understand what I have been through because at my fingertips is a group of friends who do understand. Friends who are normal broken just like me.

The clouds begin to peel away from the full moon an inch at a time. You can feel your werewolf rising within you. Where are you? Where in your body do you feel your change into werewolf form starting?

Have you been able to connect with someone who is broken in a similar way to you? Who are they and what is it about them that brings you comfort or, at the very least, helps you to feel a little more normal broken?

If these prompts don't connect with you, feel free to write about anything that does.

9

When Your Grief Becomes Destructive

Not so deep down, we all know that safety is an illusion, that only character melds us together. That's why most of us do everything we can (healthy and unhealthy) to ward off that real feeling of standing alone so close to the edge of the world.

—Kiese Laymon

Aside from bug bites and zits, few things get better when we ignore them. So, it makes sense that a first step to healing would simply be to express our grief. Maybe this seems ridiculous because your grief is all-consuming: it comes on with little warning, and when it passes, you're left feeling like you've been exorcised. But for others, it can be easier to shove grief under a couch cushion to be dealt with later. There is a to-do list that needs to be accomplished and people to be strong for, leaving no time for exorcising dark emotions. Been there, I get it. The thing is, expressing grief is only the *first* step; then we have to process it. Honestly, it is no wonder that grief is exhausting—it is so much freaking work to just get out of bed, then grief goes and asks us to think about it, too? Way harsh, Tai.

Expressing grief can take many forms, from daily naps to possessed sobbing and all the steps in between. What's important is that it is experienced—it is felt. This may look different for each person (see chapter four), and that's okay! But we must acknowledge, accept, and feel it. Look, grief sucks, but it doesn't get less sucky when you shove it into some dark corner. It will only fester, turn sour, and stink up your entire life. Painful? Yes. Scary? Yes. Uncomfortable? Also yes.

But because I am stubborn, I had to learn the hard way just how volcanically destructive suppressing grief can be. In the months after Adelaide passed away, I filled my schedule with travel and events—anything to stay in motion. An object in motion is more likely to stay in motion, and I was terrified that if I stopped, I would never get going again. Or at least that's what I told myself and those close to me. In reality, I was terrified of facing her absence, of being in a home where she would never be again, of having to sit down for regular meals as a family of three. The longer I stayed busy, the longer I could put off facing our new reality and all the pain that came with it.

My denial of how Adelaide's loss was affecting me must have been glaringly evident to everyone except, of course, me. But then the COVID-19 pandemic swept through our lives, and the world hit pause. There was nowhere left to run, I was trapped, and the stillness finally caught up to me with the power of an out-of-control freight train. I was utterly derailed.

Our once-bustling house, filled with the beeps of her machines, comings and goings of nurses and therapists, and ever-present whooshing and wheezing of her oxygen concentrator, had fallen eerily silent. Sitting on our couch, overseeing Jackson's virtual second-grade learning, I heard sounds in our building that I had never noticed before: our neighbor's dog barking, someone taking a shower, the buzz of the intercom when someone had food delivered. Every clatter, babble, or din was a reminder of the absence of the noise that surrounded Adelaide during her life.

In April 2020, barely one month into lockdown, the pressure reached a boiling point when I "celebrated" my thirty-eighth birthday. My dearest friends in Chicago ordered a rather large and slightly garish smiley-face balloon display, which was assembled on the fence outside our condo window. I met them on the sidewalk and we social distanced in homemade masks while drinking mimosas out of plastic cups. But the party didn't stop for me when everyone went home. Nope, for the rest of the day I continued to drink whatever was in arm's reach, hoping to blur out my grief in a continuous drunken haze. It worked: I had a great day . . . from what I remember.

The next day, not so much.

That day just happened to mark six months without Adelaide, and that detail weighed heavier than the case of wine I had attempted to drink my way through the day before—or the hangover that accompanied said case. Or the fact that I couldn't remember large chunks of the day, including interactions with Jackson, Miguel, or phone calls with friends and family. Getting blackout drunk, in the middle of the day, in front of my seven-year-old son, was not a life highlight. Basically, what I'm saying is that the early days of thirty-eight were filled with rainbows, sunshine, and cupcake-pooping unicorns.

At the time, I was fairly certain that being forced to grieve during a pandemic where I was shut off from the world, friends, family, and distractions was the next cruel phase of my trauma. But in hindsight (ugh, why does hindsight always have to be so right—like your mom, or that one friend who is *never* wrong but you hate to admit it), I'm able to see the time it afforded me as some sort of bizarre white elephant gift: at first it's just taking up space on the shelf, but then ends up being surprisingly useful. The abundance and stillness of time provided me with the space I needed to begin processing my grief.

There is a difference between suppressing your grief (drinking your way through your birthday), expressing your grief (having a tear-fueled exorcism), and processing your grief. The first two can feel out of control, like something is being done to you. Conversely, when you're processing the grief—taking it apart, analyzing the why, the when, the how instead of pushing it down or manically exploding—it becomes something you can own. Suppressing and expressing have their own place and time, but until the processing begins, grief will gravitate toward destruction like a toddler to a block tower.

Getting handsy with uppers or downers isn't the only way our grief can become destructive. It can also damage our relationships. Like when we lean into being a recluse or lash out over trivial matters.

I don't remember where my mother and I were going, but I had insisted on driving us there. It was my first time behind the wheel since Adelaide had died, and I had assured my mother repeatedly that I was fine. As I pulled out of our Chicago alley and onto the main street in front of our apartment building, I saw something catch the light as it swung into my peripheral vision. I glanced up at the source and felt every single one of my emotions simultaneously ignite in my chest.

"Mom, I need you to take the handicap placard off the rearview mirror," I asked, unable to hide the edge in my voice. My mother was looking at something on her phone.

"Okay, honey," she said, still looking at her phone.

With each passing second the emotional fire grew. After a whole five seconds I thought I might be overtaken by the flames.

"MOM! NOW!" I yelled. My lungs and my heart were at odds as my breath constricted and my heart lurched forward.

Calmly, Mom reached up to unhook the dangling placard. "Where would you like me to put it?"

"I don't care! Away! I—I just can't look at it!" I grabbed it from her hand and threw it on the floor at her feet. We weren't even two blocks from home and I had already allowed my emotions to completely engulf me and threaten to take out those around me.

Mom sat in shock for a few moments. "Was that necessary?"

"I just couldn't look at it!"

As I tried to find the words to defend my actions, the fire within me began to fizzle. The vacuum left in its wake was quickly filled by guilt and shame.

Confession: I am a recovering type A control freak who loathes when unwelcome emotions overtake my rational thoughts. *Please let me hold it together until I am in a more convenient place and time for feelings.*

Grief, though, doesn't give a rat's ass about convenience, and is incredibly difficult to control. But it can be understood. *If* you put in the effort. I know that sounds miserable—it *is* miserable; you're depleted—but processing and understanding grief is worth it.

Processing grief is more intentional than suppressing or expressing it; it is more drawn out, but has a more rewarding payoff. Processing is sitting in our grief and truly thinking about it—and I'm not talking about just throwing another bandage on the wound. I'm talking about inspecting it, cleaning it out, and making sure there aren't any extra bits of dirt stuck in there. Then throwing some ointment on it to prevent further infection, *and then* going back and redressing it over and over and over again.

As discussed in chapter five, this can be done by putting our grief into words, be it through talking to someone, writing about it, or verbally mulling it over during an excessively long and exceedingly hot shower. I cannot overstate how much power there is in language, in confining our grief to it. Unchallenged grief is amorphous and unwieldy. Defining it can loosen its grip on our lives, yes, but it can do even more. It has been proven that language has the power to heal pain, not just mask it or distract from it like some of our vices.[15] Psychologist James Pennebaker has been researching this phenomenon for years. He's found that when we share our personal experiences, whether in verbal or written form, we can find greater perspective and understanding about traumatic events, which allows us to feel better.[16]

During one study, Pennebaker asked students to write for fifteen minutes every day for four days about something painful that had occurred in their life. He noted that after only four days, the students reported feeling better, that the writing had been meaningful, and it had even improved their physical health. Words may be made of mere letters or sounds, but meaning gives them purpose and power.

It boils down to the amygdala in our brain, which is responsible for experiencing emotions. When we label our emotions, there is a reduction in amygdala activation.[17] Instead, our frontal and temporal lobes, which handle language and meaning and are also responsible for making us logical people, are activated. Basically, by putting words to our grieving emotions, we can go from irrational panic attacks to rational, meaningful thought, which sounds a lot less painful if you ask me.

We can make this literal mental shift by doing something as simple as talking through one specific trauma trigger or memory with a friend, or as involved as an hours-long, soul-scraping heart-to-heart with a mental health professional. Sometimes it's just the beginnings of a thought that is needling you, but putting it into words out loud for someone else to hear makes it real and gets the processing ball rolling.

Take that explosive moment with my mom in the car. I knew that my rage had little to do with Mom not taking the placard down fast enough. But it would take time alone, painfully reliving and writing about the moment, to understand that my anger was fueled by how I was forced to accept that we no longer needed the disability sign. That my disabled child would never travel by car again, that I could no longer lay claim to this widely known symbol and corresponding community. Which itself is ridiculous because I cried when I received our first placard, not wanting to accept that we needed it. These emotional contradictions had only been kerosene on the already temperamental fire churning inside me.

In the years following Adelaide's death, writing, whether for public or private consumption, became my go-to processing tool of choice. Privately, I keep a journal where the entries are addressed to Adelaide. I don't force myself to write in it daily—only when the mood strikes or when there is something I wish she was here to experience or a question I wish she could answer. Then, publicly, I have my weekly blog. However, you should know that by the time my grief processing becomes widely Googleable, I've talked about it, written about it, and edited it at length. It may seem raw to everyone else, but in reality, it has already been washed, treated, and re-bandaged several times. I say this for several reasons: first off, my first drafts are never as clean or rational as what is publicly posted, but also because it's all part of my grief processing process. When I edit something I've written, I'm ingraining those emotions into my memory. I'm questioning and analyzing. I'm reading as an outsider and making sure my thoughts are clear, not just for someone else, but for me as well.

By putting pen to paper, or fingers to keys, I can begin to own the emotions—to move them from my amygdala to my frontal lobe where I am better able to contain them. I build paragraphs around understanding different aspects of my grief, and then, once I've reread my words and accepted their illogicalities and truths, I can put that piece of my grief to the side. It doesn't disappear, necessarily, but it's not nearly as painful. Then the cool thing about the written word is that, if or when the pain resurfaces, I can always go back and reread conclusions I've already come to and solutions I've already found. Writing lets anyone become their very own grief guide, which is something the independent and stubborn sides of my personality find particularly satisfying.

It's sort of like having some kind of self-healing superpower—except instead of physical healing, it's emotional healing. I mean, if I got to choose a superpower it would probably be the ability to teleport. You'd never have to miss a holiday with family, could get away to exotic locations whenever you wanted, and could practically be in two places at once, though I suppose I would no longer be able to come up with an excuse for why I can't be somewhere when the truth is I just have no desire to go . . . okay, I may need to rethink this. I digress. But even though self-healing isn't the power *I* would have chosen, it's the one I need. When our grief becomes destructive to ourselves and/or others, transferring those emotions from the amygdala to the frontal lobe is one way we can help ourselves heal.

Writing has helped me work through my expressive grief as well, particularly those times when I don't know what has caused an emotional meltdown, because let's face it: sometimes they erupt with little warning or obvious cause. I'll write about the meltdown itself, what it feels like physically, what I see around me, what I hear in the silence after I've calmed. Even just writing about the sensory experience can bring me a sense of peace and control that I wouldn't otherwise have. If I'm out of the house or in the middle of something and have a grief revelation, I'll take a moment to jot it down in the Notes app of my phone so that I can remember to talk or write about it later (and then hope that it still makes sense to future me).

Whether through conversation or writing, the path forward necessitates that we get our feelings out of our head and into the world. If you don't work to understand your grief, then your possessed sobbing sessions will keep hitting you, it will remain easier to reach for a bottle than a keyboard, and you may end up pushing away the people you so desperately need to listen as you word vomit your longing, regrets, and pain.

Take it at your own pace—a trickle over time or a torrential watershed, entirely up to you. No matter how you process, what I can tell you is that it will be continuous. I doubt that I'll ever stop processing. There will always be something new to work through because our grief shape-shifts over time—different parts of life will push different emotional bruises with more focused intensity or not at all. The hardest part, though, as is true with most things in life, is just getting started. Making the choice to feel better, process, and eventually, heal.

Write about the last time your grief pushed you until you felt out of control. Where were you? What were you doing? Can you pinpoint what set your grief off? What could you smell, hear, see? What did you feel physically?

I challenge you to choose one aspect of your grief and write about it for ten minutes every day for a week.

If these prompts don't connect with you, feel free to write about anything that does.

_____

_____

_____

_____

_____

_____

_____

_____

_____

_____

_____

_____

_____

_____

_____

_____

10

When You're Not Sure If You Want to Heal

> The heart is an instrument, once broken, never repairs the same. I use the word "trauma" in my work, because a loss is a loss, whether it's a heart, a limb, a promise, a person. It's all loss, and it's all trauma, and it's all things that are broken that can't be cured. You can't go back. But you can heal it, and that's an important thing to know.
>
> —Kevin Kling

In the last few years, there have been few among us that haven't shouldered grief they had previously thought unimaginable, unbearable, even insurmountable. Grief is not, actually, any of those things—it's just more pain than we've ever had to overcome before. Because deep grief is so misunderstood until it is experienced firsthand, it is not uncommon to hear "advice" that sounds something like, "You could choose to be happy again if you would just move on with your life." As if grieving the emotional and/or physical loss of a person is the equivalent of pouting. It doesn't help that our society tries to get us to rush through the less attractive grieving stages and get right into the more Instagrammable healing ones with our face turned toward the perfectly angled sunlight.

Raises hand. Guilty!

So, it should come as no surprise that I grew to despise the thought of healing.

Every few months, my mom would send me another book on healing from grief that I would add to the growing pile next to my bed. I would look at them each night before bed, but couldn't bring myself to open a cover, let alone read their contents. And no, the irony of me going on to write a similar book is not lost on me. But I guess that's why this book is now here, because those books assumed from the start that I had a desire to heal, and while outwardly I said I just wasn't ready, it's closer to the truth to say that I didn't want to. While no one ever explicitly said to me that it was time to "get over it," that was the subtext I attached to healing. I also couldn't fathom a way to move on from such all-consuming pain without somehow not remembering it. Not remembering Adelaide. Maybe moving on didn't mean forgetting exactly, but it meant letting go in some way, or not looking back. And that was *not* going to work for me.

I know I am not alone in desperately needing to remember because, among other things, I'm not alone in getting a tribute tattoo inked on my body. Many of us in grief permanently mark our bodies—not just to memorialize our person, but so that we are continuously reminded of them every time we catch the ink out of the corner of our eye. It is also a visible statement for others to bear witness to so that they might remember. It's a pretty intense testimony when you think about it.

Permanent ink will remind us of the essence of our person, but the crap thing is that our memories of them fade no matter how hard we try to hold on to them. A phrase they once said becomes jumbled, the lyrics to a special lullaby grow fuzzy, and did we go on that vacation before or after I started the new job? I certainly didn't need healing to come along and speed up this unavoidable process.

Sure, photos, videos, and journals can help solidify a memory, but they can't capture the way Adelaide felt in my lap when I held her. The weight of her body. The listlessness of her head, too heavy for her hypotonic muscles to manage on their own. The near-gravitational pull of her thumb to her mouth until the seizures took her ability to coordinate that movement as well. The way her eyes rolled to look at me and the smell of her freshly washed hair, which lingered for days because she rarely left our home for more than a stroller walk. Photos will help me remember our trip to Disney World, but it is the responsibility of my mind alone to hold on to the feeling of her entire hand gripping my thumb so that I wouldn't leave her side at bedtime.

And then underlying all my misgivings about what healing looked like was my belief that I did not *deserve* to heal. That my pain was a sort of penance for surviving when my daughter didn't. How dare I heal when she never could? All of these thoughts and feelings combined to create an acrimonious aversion to healing.

That is, until I heard five words that forever changed the trajectory of my healing journey:

"To heal, we must remember."

President Joe Biden spoke these words at a COVID-19 remembrance ceremony the night before his inauguration. I was struck by their simplicity, their truth, and the hope they inspired. Here was someone telling me that my healing journey *didn't* mean moving on and leaving the past behind me, but moving forward *while* holding on to the memories of what was. That this message came from a man who had also grieved significant losses—his wife and infant daughter in a car accident, then decades later his adult son to brain cancer—and yet had survived, persevered, and achieved more than most, helped it reach me with an unexpected clarity. I mean, regardless of your political affiliation, you have to agree that the man certainly knows a thing or two about grieving.

Around this time, my mother sent me a text checking in, ever concerned about my emotional well-being: "It takes a lot of work to get yourself unstuck and you're weary. Grief is emotionally and physically exhausting. It's easy to stay in your warm little cocoon . . . but now is a great time to help yourself and look to the future with hope."

She was right; I was stuck. My disinterest in healing had turned me into a high-functioning griever: I no longer spent a majority of my time in the dark, but I was still regularly fighting the temptation to slip back toward that shell. And when I found myself there yet again, I convinced myself that I was comfortable in my cocoon. Sure, it was incredibly dark and cramped and closed off from the world, but I'd made a home there, with decorative pillows, plush throws, and cozy rugs. I also knew that in order to break out of this cycle, I'd have to make an intense effort. I've never been afraid of difficult work, though I have undoubtedly suffered from a lack of motivation, direction, and self-worth. But until I heard President Biden's words, I didn't understand what kind of work healing would be. It isn't difficult because I'd have to let go of my grief and move on; it is difficult because I have to live with it and still move forward.

In some ways, this is bizarrely comforting. Knowing that the grief will always be with me means I don't have to worry about losing it, or, rather, losing this piece of Adelaide that remains. If you lost your arm in a horrible accident, you would never forget what it was like having an arm, but you would learn to function without it. In many ways, this is similar—except instead of a limb, we've lost a chunk of our heart. It's why we create memorials after mass casualty events or place plaques on park benches. Remembering *is* healing.

Okay, so if healing could be about remembering, then maybe, *maybe*, I was willing to give it a try. After all, I had to admit that sometimes I did want to scoot away from my dark precipice, to not be constantly peering over its edge. I did want to break free of the depression that sucked away my energy and tempted me with meaningless distraction. I wanted to disband the anxiety that congregated in my chest, claiming to be on the lookout for emotional provocateurs, but actually creating a chronic state of disquiet. I wasn't convinced yet that I deserved to, but still . . .

To heal, we must remember.

But where to start? Life has a funny way of presenting you with a path when you decide upon a direction, and this time was no exception. Since Adelaide's death, I had noticed a flare in my grief-induced anxiety whenever I was away from home and felt like something was taking too long—whether that was standing in a checkout line, waiting for the pharmacist to fill a prescription, or even just casually conversing at a social gathering. I'm not sure how to describe it other than as an extreme fight or flight response that took over my entire mind and body, telling me I needed to go home. Typically, once I was headed home, the feeling subsided and I forgot about it entirely. Sometimes, though, it would take a nap or medication to mute this primal alarm.

Then one day, not long after I had decided to give healing a try, I made myself remember. I'd had a flare of anxiety in the grocery, but made it safely to the parking lot. My heart rate was easing, and, instead of trying to block out the uncomfortable experience, I tried to figure out what had triggered the attack. Yes, the line had been long, but I had been up next when the pressure began to build. Also, there was nothing I needed to rush home for . . . not anymore.

And so I remembered.

A couple years before, we had only recently made the excruciating decision to begin hospice services for Adelaide, and I was emotionally drained and in need of a temporary distraction. I had just finished a workout class and let myself be talked into going to a matinee movie with friends. We thought we still had months with Adelaide. She'd been stable that morning and our home nurse was with her—she was in incredibly capable hands.

On the way home from the movie, I got a call from Adelaide's nurse that her breath rate and oxygen levels had plummeted. Without intervention, she would need resuscitation soon—and only days before, I had signed the "Do Not Resuscitate" form.

"Would you like me to intervene?" her nurse asked me.

I wasn't ready to make the decision to let Adelaide go, to say goodbye. I needed more time. "Yes . . . yes! I'll be right there."

After that, for the next four weeks, I didn't leave Adelaide's side until she left mine forever.

Trauma with a capital T and that rhymes with G and that stands for grief, gloom, or guilt—take your pick. (Now that my musical theater–adept readers have *The Music Man* cast recording stuck in their heads . . .) Anyway, I think I've identified why what appeared to be impatience on steroids was actually my trauma manifesting in a stress response. Maybe remembering wasn't just about holding on to the best moments, but acknowledging those I had repressed as well. These specific panic attacks had a deeply rooted, if currently irrational, motivator. I could heal that trauma, and the associated grief, by remembering it (not dwelling on it; remembering and dwelling are two separate actions)—by recognizing that it had occurred, that it was a part of the way I now processed the world around me.

This isn't to say that our grief is something to overcome. It's not an enemy we need to battle and vanquish. It's more like a companion that may or may not always be welcome, but remains a companion all the same. It's up to us to frame what kind of companion it is, how we view it, and how we live with it. And, to President Biden's point, how we remember it.

To heal, we must remember.

While I had suppressed *this* specific memory, it is not uncommon for me to dwell on my more negative memories, questioning what I could have done differently. After all, while we are surviving grief it can be easier to sit in some of our heavier memories: those filled with fear, regret, and mourning more closely match the pain we are internalizing.

Then there's the basic science of it. Researchers have determined that negative emotional events in particular activate the part of our brain responsible for boosting memory.[18] Essentially, evolution has hardwired our brains to remember negative memories more vividly than positive ones so that we remember potential dangers or sensitive settings in the future and, ideally, avoid them. Great for avoiding extinction, not so much for maintaining our emotional well-being.

The last thing I'll say about spending too much time in the dark space may come off as a bit harsh, but here it is: grief is a selfish emotion. Now, this does not mean that it doesn't need to be felt and expressed. Clearly, it does. (Otherwise, I wouldn't have written an entire book about it!) But it is undeniably self-serving. The simple, rational truth is that my pain doesn't benefit Adelaide. It won't bring her back, and I'm fairly certain she is not looking down on me in judgment, evaluating whether I am grieving her enough. Pain only begets more pain, and by punishing myself, by depriving myself of healing, I am only hurting myself and those I love most. I say this not to make anyone feel guilty for expressing their grief, but because it's important to recognize that our grief and healing can coexist. And, perhaps more importantly, to recognize that we deserve to heal.

You deserve to heal.

And to heal, we must remember.

The negative and traumatic memories aren't going anywhere—and we may not want them to. They happened and are a part of us now—but that doesn't mean that they need to pull focus. Again, dwelling and remembering are not the same. This means we must hold space for the happy memories as well, to remind ourselves of what joy feels like so we can work toward experiencing it again. Because, contrary to what our guilt may tell us, we do truly deserve to be happy.

It was one of those brilliant late-spring days where you bring a jacket with you out of habit, but quickly abandon it for the vitamin D radiating from the heavens. Jackson had soccer practice at a nearby park, and instead of dropping him off and leaving to run errands, I decided to sit with a book and enjoy the weather. Toward the end of his practice, a woman stepped out of her suburban-family, standard-issue, three-row SUV (the new millennium's comeback to the wood-paneled minivan of my youth). We locked eyes for a moment, and, inspired by the warmth of the day, I abandoned my grief-driven reclusive tendencies and smiled at her. She immediately smiled back and began walking in my direction.

Shit! What had I done? I didn't speak to people and certainly not strangers.

"Hi! Which one is yours?" She asked pointing to the gaggle of boys running amok on the field.

"Jackson, in the red shirt."

"Oh! You're Jackson's mom! We met your husband a few weeks ago. I'm Alex's mom. It's so nice to meet you."

We chatted for a few minutes about our boys before I pushed the conversation toward the uncomfortable to take control and get it out of the way.

"Do you have other children?" I asked.

"Yep, two little girls: six and two. What about you?"

"A daughter, Adelaide. She passed away a couple years ago from a neuro-degenerative condition and epilepsy just before her fourth birthday. It was basically as awful as it sounds and still sucks *a lot*, but we're managing."

Alex's mom had the same look of pity and sorrow that I had grown accustomed to, but what came out of her mouth next flattened me:

"What was she like?"

No stranger had ever asked me that before. I was typically met with guilt and uncomfortable silence, sometimes even a physical step backward. But this woman had leaned in, not with morbid curiosity about her illness or death, but interested in who Adelaide was as a person.

Sitting on that park bench with Alex's mom, talking about Adelaide's favorite books and music, I felt a small crack in my heart fill in. I had been so terrified of having to recount the most painful echoes of Adelaide's life with strangers that I'd forgotten that I could also talk about the ones that bring me laughter, energy, and joy. Sharing the details of her personality, likes, and life was the opposite of traumatic. It was a salve. Sharing her memory—remembering—was healing.

I now see that I need to honor both my positive and negative memories if I want to heal, each getting their share. The trickiest part of healing by remembering may be finding this balance. No one wants to be known as a person with a lot of baggage, yet it is from that "baggage"—our hardest trials—that we derive and fortify our strength. What a tragedy it would be to disregard all I've learned from my life's challenging moments because I don't want to acknowledge past pain. Also, those not-as-pleasant memories don't just disappear because I'm not focusing on them. I can tie them to an anchor and throw them into the depths of my subconscious, but they are still tethered to me, waiting for the most inconvenient moment to resurface. Like while standing in line at the grocery store, for instance.

While we only have so much control over the number of bags we are saddled with, what we can control is how we manage and remember them. These memories may appear to be constructs of the past, but I've found that it's a bad idea to underestimate their power to shape the future. As I share my memories of Adelaide, I recognize that I am ultimately responsible for constructing how she is remembered in the present and in the future. Which memories and characteristics do I want to float to the top?

And questioning that then got me wondering, how do I want to be remembered? Not as a mother who lost her child and lived in debilitating grief forever after. I want to be remembered as a woman who fought for her child and then went on to fight for others, who loved deeply, laughed loudly, and shared generously. Likewise, I don't want Adelaide to be remembered solely as a child who suffered and died. This is part of her story, but is not her whole story. She was also a brave and resilient little girl who clung to life, warmed the heart of every person she met, and loved a good snuggle right up until she didn't.

Elisabeth Kübler-Ross, who pioneered the idea of the stages of grief (see chapter six), wrote, "The most beautiful people we have known are those who have known defeat, known suffering, known struggle, known loss, and have found their way out of the depths. These persons have an appreciation, a sensitivity, and an understanding of life that fills them with compassion, gentleness, and a deep loving concern. Beautiful people do not just happen."[19]

Beautiful people do not just happen.

They are broken and forcefully remolded, they are chiseled away at and sanded down, they are put through the fire and run over the coals—and yet they continue to survive. Would they rather not have gone through all of that? I'm sure! I know I wish I hadn't. But I am undeniably stronger and an altogether better person for having experienced trauma, grief, and loss. I am a better person for having known Adelaide. This is the energy we need to move forward, and we can do it *while* remembering those we've loved and lost. In fact, in order for that poignantly earned beauty to endure, it is imperative that we remember them.

Yes, first you have to make the choice to heal, but please know that you are capable and you deserve to. Allow yourself to become one of those beautiful people. Because healing isn't cutting ties and forgetting. It's persevering and remembering.

How do you want to be remembered?

How do you want to remember your loved ones?

How would they want to be remembered?

If these prompts don't connect with you, feel free to write about anything that does.

_____

_____

_____

_____

_____

_____

_____

_____

_____

_____

_____

_____

_____

_____

_____

11

When Gratitude Is a Struggle

> In our culture I think most people think of grief as sadness, and that's certainly part of it, a large part of it, but there's also this thorniness, these edges that come out.
>
> —Anthony Rapp

It wasn't until I had experienced the life-shattering effects of grief that I grasped just how unsettling toxic positivity, and its close cousin forced gratitude, could be. I got a taste of these during Adelaide's life while charting a course through her medical complexities. But even then (especially then?) I clung to hope for Adelaide's well-being like Rose floating on the wooden door in *Titanic*, even as she watched the life she had envisioned for herself slip below the surface of the water with her beloved Jack.

In those early day's following Adelaide's first seizures, I desperately clung to the idea of silver linings, collecting and stringing them together to show to anyone who looked at me with sorrow or pity. They were the lifelong friendships made within a community we never would have otherwise met. They were the sense of purpose and drive I found while raising awareness and money for poorly funded epilepsy research. They were the pride I found in knowing my daughter better than anyone else and advocating fiercely for her best interests. However, after countless seizures, meds, side effects, and near-death experiences, it became harder and harder to find even a sliver of good amidst all the pain. Yet even in those final months, even with their glint dulled, I still found silver linings in our quietest moments: momentary eye contact that told me Adelaide knew I was there with her, a squeeze of my finger, and every last snuggle.

After her death, color faded from my world, shapes blended, time blurred. I had no use for silver linings, nothing left to hope for. But, wow, did people feel the need to make sure I knew they were still there!

"At least she's no longer suffering."
"At least your son is healthy."
"At least you won't have to spend time at the hospital anymore."

As Dr. Brené Brown so notably said, "Rarely, if ever, does an empathic response begin with 'at least.'" As far as I'm concerned, the combination of those two words together—and the meaning they imply—should be stricken from all human language, altogether, forever. Because even if the sentiments didn't begin with 'at least,' they might as well have.

"Look at all the lives she touched."
"See all the good you made happen in her honor!"

None of these replies were wrong, which made my aggressive resistance to peace offerings that much more confusing to me. Seriously, outside of my profoundly significant loss, my life is pretty amazing. I remember walking around a bustling Christmas market two months after Adelaide passed, clinging to my steaming cider for warmth, watching Jackson stare in wonder at a booth stacked to its squat rafters with glittering snow globes, all that holiday magic reflecting off his schoolboy face.

How fortunate was I to be able to celebrate the holidays with my family? *But it's not my whole family . . .*

How fortunate was I to be able to afford to have plentiful gifts under the tree? *But there wouldn't be any for Adelaide this year . . .*

I had so much to be thankful for! Why was I letting this one loss, this one exception to my good fortune tear me apart? At the same time, I wanted to scream that I would trade all the good to have Adelaide alive and healthy. Or, in my darkest moments, that I would gladly have the suffering Adelaide back just to have more time with her. They could keep their silver linings, their "at leasts," and all the rest of their positive musings. I would just like my daughter back.

There is no point in trying to reconcile all we have with what we've lost. There is no master tally sheet or referee keeping score. Perhaps if you believe in karma and reincarnation then it will all come out in the wash in our next life, but there is no guarantee that our dealt hand balances out in *this* earthly lifetime—and if it does, according to who? Trying to mentally balance these scales is wasted effort when energy is already sparse. Additionally, attempts to do so, along with sentiments like "Look at all you have to be thankful for," take the focus off of what's been lost. And *that* can feel like people are diminishing our grief, or at minimum shoving it aside, when all we want to do—when all we *can* do—is cling to it and remember. It can feel almost patronizing, like an adult trying to distract a toddler from crying over a scraped knee with a lollipop. These situations can be especially present and challenging around the winter holidays, when everywhere you look, from Facebook posts to Hallmark Christmas movies, reminds you to be grateful. What kind of horrible person was I if I couldn't find and hold on to end-of-year gratitude?

Grief and gratitude have a deeply complicated relationship: our grief is more intense when we have the most gratitude for what we've lost. Gratitude for every day I had with my daughter is at the very root of my grief, because I know that what I am most thankful for, I will never have again in this life. It is not that we are ungrateful—it is that gratitude can bring as much pain as it does joy.

When silver linings go from being a source of hope to one of searing pain, they've crossed the threshold into forced gratitude, a close cousin of the much-admonished toxic positivity. This is not to say that we shouldn't have gratitude for all the good in our lives—we absolutely should. Focusing on the good helps drive us forward and lift our spirits. Gratitude on its own is an incredibly powerful motivator, pushing us to give back and maintain a sense of positivity. But the problems occur when it becomes a false sense of positivity—when the gratitude is used to force negative emotions down.

We can absolutely be grateful that we have our health, or a surviving child, or a supportive family, or a remaining parent, but the second our gratitude for them is tied to strife, trauma, or loss, we are unwittingly sowing the seeds of guilt and resentment in the very soil from which we are hoping to cultivate growth. We don't have to be grateful for something or someone *because* we have lost something else. The loss taints the gratitude; it becomes forced, and instead of being a motivator for good, it weighs us down with confusion. Because we should be grateful, right? Sure, our loved one is gone, and this is nowhere near the life we had envisioned for ourselves or them, but those "at least" statements aren't wrong . . . Shouldn't our losses make us that much more appreciative of the good?

Potentially unpopular opinion here, but I'm going to give that question a resounding "Nope." I don't require the death of one child to make me extra grateful for my living child. Nor does the fact that I have a living child make my loss any less painful. It is not my responsibility to validate someone else's need to find some sort of cosmic balance as they witness my pain. Relieve yourself of the weight of that guilt, of that forced gratitude.

Hiding between the folds of forced gratitude is comparative grief, and, in its most toxic form, competitive grief. We can strain and reach, trying to find purpose in either, but neither have a space at the healthy grieving table, and both need to be pulled out at their roots like the invasive weeds they are.

After Adelaide passed, I was introduced to a family who had also recently lost a child. Their son had passed overnight from a seizure, a condition called Sudden Unexpected Death in Epilepsy, or SUDEP. He had been in elementary school, and was otherwise healthy, developmentally typical, and had a bright future ahead of him. Unlike Adelaide's loss, his death had been a shock to their family.

Following a conversation between the dads, Miguel lamented to me that he'd had a difficult time connecting about their mutual losses with the boy's father. We'd had a years-long runway to prepare for Adelaide's altered and eventually shortened future. Whether or not we liked to admit it, her final exhale came with some relief. Both our families had lost a child, and both charged epilepsy with, if not being the perpetrator, at least as an accessory to the crime. Yet our grieving journeys were miles apart from each other.

"I told him I couldn't imagine losing a seemingly healthy child, that you knew so well and had plans with and for. How awful.

"And then he said to me that he couldn't imagine never truly knowing his child."

Oof.

This conversation comes to mind whenever I sense the urge to compare grief poking up through the surface of my subconscious. As someone once told me, comparison may be the thief of joy, but it is also the thief of grief. There is no better or worse way to lose someone. Sudden or anticipated, it all seriously sucks. They both have their trauma and accompanying therapy bills, yet somehow we are still drawn to this inane competition. Either we are trying to diminish our own grief by seeing someone else's as more significant, or we are trying to bolster our grief, to give it more weight by diminishing someone else's.

Why, though? To what end?

Deciding that my circumstance is not as heavy as someone else's has *never* made me feel better. Conversely, there is no award for who has endured the most. I can understand how it could be validating to compare our pain to someone else's and decide that it is significant or profound enough to be exacting the toll that it is—but that's diminishing someone else's loss to benefit my battered psyche. It is like the ultimate "at least" statement, an unnecessary body slam on an already injured teammate.

There is no grief hierarchy. Losing a parent is no easier or harder than losing a grandparent, which is no easier or harder than losing a spouse. I couldn't even fathom a guess as to how many times someone has said to me that their loss doesn't come close to what I experienced losing a child. As if child loss is the grief holy grail. We are not the master arbiters of a loss's effect on anyone's life but our own, which means that everyone's grief is valid, regardless of how we think it would affect us. We can empathize and hold space with another person without pulling rank. In fact, the moment we begin to judge and rank is the moment our empathy becomes false.

Grief is shaped by a lifetime of lived experiences: what the person means to us, all the ways they were connected to us, the stability or fragility of the relationship during life and especially at the end, the responsibility or lack thereof that they leave us with, our physical and mental health at the time of the loss. So many factors go into how a loss impacts us. Perspective is everything, and there are no unilateral criteria or objective standards by which grief can be measured. So let it be subjective. Let yourself listen to and be there for someone else's journey. Let their grief stand apart from your own.

In certain situations, we can find relief and answers by flexing the power of the word "and," by drawing on our ability to hold two conflicting emotions in our heads and hearts at the same time. Instead of forcing one to win out, hold them both simultaneously: acknowledge your pain AND also be grateful, acknowledge someone else's pain AND also your own. You can be excited that your brother is getting married to an amazing person AND sad that your parent isn't alive to witness it. You can be thrilled that your child got into their dream college AND sorely miss your spouse as you celebrate. You can wish your child hadn't suffered during their brief life AND be there for a friend whose child was lost unexpectedly. Hold space and give time to both/all the feelings. By not forcing the grief down or comparing it to others', we can allow ourselves to still be present for life's more enjoyable moments while also maintaining much-needed relationships. Life is complicated and emotions are contradictory, but that doesn't make any of them false. It simply means they all need their moment, and living with "and" can make that happen.

Recently, though, I've recognized that sometimes "and" isn't enough. Two years and two weeks after Adelaide passed away, we received a call about a two-and-a-half-year-old little girl in Texas who was in need of a family. The call was about as out of the blue as they come. As if this child was falling from the sky and into our arms.

"Are we actually doing this? Are we really about to pick up a child who will one day be our daughter?"

"I think we are," Miguel answered me with wonder and caution.

It all happened so quickly. We got the call on Monday, and by Friday we were driving away from a CPS office in Texas with a child we had never met in the backseat of our rental car. Given my tendency to overanalyze, I know the quick turnaround was for the best. Truthfully, there were only twenty-four hours to prepare since I wouldn't let myself get my hopes up that this was indeed happening. Any number of issues could have arisen preventing this little girl from coming into our lives, and I was terrified of having this dream dashed.

That turnaround meant the day before we flew to Dallas was a busy one. Jackson and I made a pit stop at Target for essentials: pajamas and several outfits in multiple sizes because we didn't know how big she was, sippy cups, activities for the plane ride, and an enormous Minnie Mouse stuffed animal that Jackson picked out personally.

The biggest adjustment, though, was making space in our home because it meant Adelaide had to, in a sense, move out. When we moved back to New Jersey, it had been important to me that Adelaide have a room in our new home. She would never live in it, obviously, but I wanted her to have a space where any of us could go to feel close to her. The room doubled as my office, a guest room, and the place I ran to when I needed a quiet space to scream into a pillow and drown in my own tears.

Art created in her memory, along with a framed scrap of wallpaper from her Chicago bedroom, adorned the walls. The IV pole that had held her feeding pump sat in the corner and was now home to the mobile that had hung over her crib, the flower crown my cousin made for her to wear at her Make-A-Wish birthday party, and some other mementos. Her favorite books were lined up on the bottom shelf of a bookcase that had once held some of her medical equipment. I had bought new bedding and hung fresh curtains so it didn't feel like a total shrine, but still, her presence there was undeniable.

But now, Anessa would need that room.

There wasn't time to redecorate for her the way I would eventually, but I wanted her to feel comfortable in the space when she arrived. I wanted her to know this room was hers and it was safe. To do that would require ignoring the myriad of emotions tied to my next actions.

I moved my desk out first, along with my personal books and office belongings. I sorted through various stuffed animals, boxing up Adelaide's favorites— in part because I didn't want anything to happen to them, but also because I got this strange feeling that Adelaide wouldn't want to share them. Which sounds bizarre but, well, that was Adelaide, and also what three-year-old wants to share their favorite stuffies?

Miguel walked in as I was taking pictures off the walls and almost immediately his eyes went glassy, in a rare show of emotion.

"If you're going to cry I need you to go somewhere else because I can't stop to think about what I'm doing. If I fall into the dark place right now, I'm not sure I will be able to climb back out," I said, refusing to make eye contact as I rolled the IV pole out into the hall.

I went down to the basement, to the massive black trunk that Miguel had been given when he was on tour with the musical *The 25th Annual Putnam County Spelling Bee* and opened it for the first time in years. Inside were Jackson's favorite toys, which I had held on to for Adelaide. I had known years earlier that Adelaide would never play with the trunk's contents, but I had never been able to bring myself to go through it. So, it had sat in storage collecting expensive dust.

I opened the heavy lid and stared at the trucks, plastic pots and pans, and wooden building blocks. Had I been holding on to these for another child of mine all along? Nope, too much emotion tied to that thought train. I pushed it all down, unable to sort through the "ands" in that moment as I carried the well-loved toys up.

A couple months later, this situation would arise again. Clothes, books, and gifts that my mom had bought for Adelaide but never been able to give her were opened by Anessa at Christmas. I was overjoyed to have Anessa in our home and our hearts, to give her a Christmas of her dreams, to cuddle her and love on her and let her unfiltered joy wash over us. AND it was entirely unfair that Adelaide wasn't here to enjoy the gifts that had been meant for her and to feel our love physically. Nothing about it was fair, no matter how much we loved—and love—them both.

I'm not sure if I've ever been so happy, depressed, grateful, and angry all at the same time. I tried to push the emotions down, to enjoy the moment, but I had run out of space. So, instead they exploded out of my face in sobs. Miguel quietly hugged me as the kids, distracted by Santa's offerings, tore into their stockings in the next room.

On this day, "and" just wasn't going to cut it. Yes, I missed Adelaide AND was grateful for Anessa. I knew that growing our family had been the right decision, the best decision. AND it was not lost on me that it was highly unlikely that Anessa would have come into our lives without Adelaide leaving. But using "and" here had me questioning if I had just replaced one daughter with another. Did being grateful for Anessa mean I was in turn grateful for Adelaide's death? Or that I should be? Because I wasn't and never could be. Was I even truly grateful for Anessa then? What if I had to choose between them? My mind swirled with conscious irrationalities, but in the height of emotions, rationality is often left defenseless.

Sometimes the path to less guilt, to fully appreciating the good—without feeling forced to—has to begin with cutting the tether between our losses and fortunes. One does not have to have anything to do with the other. I would argue that they can even be two completely different sentences—replace "and" with a period, and you are getting closer to finding a balance, or at least a coexistence.

This is not the life I envisioned.
I am grateful for the good in the life that I have.

Both statements are true. They do not need to have any correlation to each other to remain true. Yes, shitty things have happened, they sucked, and they are wildly unfair. Good things are also happening, and deep down we want to enjoy them. Not because we "should," not because of our ill-fated past, but because we deserve to enjoy and appreciate the good just for being good.

This is not the life I envisioned.
I am grateful for the good in the life that I have.
No "at least"; no "and"—just because.

We don't always have to reconcile our past with our present, our hurt with our joy. Let each stand on its own. Write about a piece of your loss that hurts a little extra today. Then, write about something you are grateful for today that you can detach from your loss.

If these prompts don't connect with you, feel free to write about anything that does.

⟶≫≫≫≻

_____

_____

_____

_____

_____

_____

_____

_____

_____

_____

_____

_____

_____

_____

12

When You Feel Emotionally Hungover

Sometimes exhaustion is not a result of too much time spent on something, but of knowing that in its place, no time is spent on something else.

—Joyce Rachelle

EMOTIONAL HANGOVER PUNCH

Ingredients

- Grief resulting from a significant loss
- One day of basic socialization
- At least an hour's worth of tears

Instructions

1. Pour ingredients into a slightly-too-small container.
2. Shake well.
3. Let sit overnight in an overactive brain.
4. Optional garnish: prior night's used tissues.

Best served with anti-depressants and cuddles in bed.

Shortly after moving from Chicago to New Jersey, I discovered just how significantly my social bandwidth had been compromised. Excited to reconnect with friends, Miguel and I made the early miscalculation to schedule a couple back-to-back visits. In the moment, I was happy to see people we hadn't seen in years, catch up, and give COVID-safe air hugs. We always discussed Adelaide because it would be weird if we didn't. Her absence was felt as strongly as a dog tugging on its leash—it was a pulling, a yearning.

But then I proceeded to spend the entire next day in bed with what I can best describe as an emotional hangover: tightness in my chest, heavy heart, foggy head, and zero motivation to do anything, using my comforter as a shield against the outside world.

My initial response to this hangover was anger and shame at my apparent weakness. Yes, talking about Adelaide's loss is draining, but so was caring for her and I didn't require a comforter cocoon then.

But that wasn't entirely true. It just looked different.

When Adelaide was alive, I took daily naps—often for just thirty minutes, but long enough to mentally recharge from the sleepless night before. There were also my weekly cryfests when I got overwhelmed by her incessant seizures or other mystery symptoms. It wasn't weakness when Adelaide was alive, and it isn't now—it's just that my emotional cocktail of choice has changed from a salt-rimmed Desperate Caregiver to an extra-sour Unimaginable Griever. One cocktail on its own won't give you a hangover, but line them up in quick succession and you're going to be hurting in the morning. As in all aspects of our lives, we must establish our boundaries. So, if I wanted to avoid future hangovers, I would need to learn my tolerance for these interactions and plan accordingly.

Do you remember the recess game "Mother, May I"? Where there's someone playing "Mother," and a line of kids are all trying to reach the Mother? Mother tells each kid in order how many steps, hops, or skips they are allowed to take forward, and the kid has to say, "Mother, may I?" after the direction or get sent back to the starting line. It's kind of like that—we are out here processing our grief, moving through life, but every once in a while we forget to ask our mind and body permission and we are sent back to the starting line.

Except this time the consequences are more severe—not quite *Squid Game*-level, but close.

With a bit of trial and emotionally painful error, I discovered I could withstand about two social interactions a week, but not in the same day or even on consecutive days. But everyone's tolerance for these interactions is going to be different, and interactions with certain people may put us over the top quicker than others. It feels like a lot to think about when your threshold for critical thinking is already compromised, but you'll be surprised how innately you already know that going over to Jane's house with her seemingly perfect family is going to hit you like a heavy-handed Long Island iced tea, while a quiet lunch out with Jane sans family can be sipped like a refreshing spritzer.

MOTHER, MAY I?
AS LONG AS YOU RESPECT YOUR TOLERANCE.

These physical and emotional check-ins go beyond our initial capacity for social interactions immediately following the loss. I have often used a packed calendar to avoid feeling, well, anything. It can feel like an excellent tactic since I tend to thrive under pressure, with a packed calendar and a prioritized to-do list. But it turns into me metaphorically driving down an interstate with bugs constantly hitting my windshield. At some point, my windshield is so full of bug guts I can't see the road anymore and I have to pull over. (I wish I could say I choose to pull over, but let's be real, when it gets that bad, it's all about self-preservation. My life's ultimate balancing accomplishment will be when I achieve the happy medium between accomplished but crazed Kelly and grounded but depressed Kelly.)

But in the years since Adelaide died, I have worked diligently to not let my windshield get so dirty—on trying to process my grief as it comes and with *real* elbow grease instead of relying solely on an exhausted pair of windshield wipers that leave bug gut streaks behind.

Though sometimes it takes more than elbow grease to get the job done, as I learned after Adelaide's second deathiversary.

When you've lost someone, anniversaries and other meaningful dates are basically the worst (see chapter fourteen). By this point, I thought I had figured out the secret to surviving these days: fill them with activities and people, and before you know it, they are over.

So, we watched videos, looked through pictures, and went sunflower picking. There were plenty of tears, but it felt active and beautiful. Five days later, on her birthday, we celebrated Adelaide with friends and family. We laughed and shared stories, and it was surprisingly enjoyable! The days had come and gone, and I survived with only a minimal hangover. But in all the activity, I hadn't noticed the bug graveyard building on my windshield. I couldn't see that I was employing the same techniques I had used to avoid the most unsettling parts of my grief years before. That is, until the week after, when our guests had left and the stillness settled over our house once again.

It wasn't as if I hadn't acknowledged her loss, then or now. In fact, I often feel like all I do is talk about her. But sometimes, what we actually need is to let the worst of our emotions wash over us. As uncomfortable as it is, as ugly as they may be, we have to express these emotions before we can rinse our windshields and get back on the road. Like some sort of miracle cleansing soul wash.

MOTHER, MAY I?
AFTER YOU CLEAN YOUR WINDSHIELD.

Sometimes respecting our tolerance and cleaning our windshields can feel like a privilege. We don't always have the time or the privacy to lock ourselves in our room and feel all the emotions. I felt this constriction acutely as our community reopened after the pandemic. The entire world had hit pause, but then suddenly we were swan diving back into the depths of our busy lives. In speaking with friends and colleagues, I found many were (like me) trying to be a bit more selective about the activities they agreed to, but it wasn't always up to us because, spoiler, there are more people in our lives that we care for beyond ourselves. So now we are back to busy lives, whether we want to be or not, and are also still grieving those we've lost. And if that wasn't enough, those people that you care for, who are crowding your calendar, might be grieving the same loss as you.

I'm not sure how many times someone would ask me how I was doing and if I was taking care of myself during Adelaide's last year. They would remind me that "you can't pour from an empty pitcher" or that "even on an airplane, we are told to put the oxygen on ourselves first before helping others." While, yes, I knew this was true, sometimes there weren't enough hours in the day to take care of me. When you're living through traumatic times *and also* are responsible for other people, what are you supposed to do? Skip out on cooking dinner so you can go have a good cry? Or maybe multi-task and cry during dinner prep? "Gee babe, the salad is tasting extra salty this evening . . ." Abandon the kids at school so you can get a massage? "Sorry kids, Mommy needed me time."

There are work and family obligations that don't always offer space for the "Mother, may I" check-ins that we need. What then?

"Then" is when it's time to suck up your pride and ask for help from one of the dozens of people who have been asking for months what they can do to help you.

From the earliest days of Adelaide's diagnosis, I had no choice but to rely on others for help. If I was in the hospital with Adelaide and Miguel was at the theater, someone had to be with Jackson. And with no family around, that meant favors from friends became the norm. Throughout Adelaide's life, I doled out IOUs like the old man on my childhood block gave out butterscotch candies. That had been new to me, as I had always preferred to do things on my own, both because I didn't want to ask for help, and because I took immense pride in being able to announce that I had completed something by myself. In adulthood, though, there are no gold stars for solo projects, or any project for that matter. What was important was that my family was cared for and their needs were met, regardless of how many people it took to make that a reality.

I tried to follow this same logic after Adelaide passed, but it wasn't always easy. I had lost the very reason I'd needed help in the first place. With so much newfound, albeit undesired, time on my hands, what was my excuse for asking now?

But that was the very problem with my thinking. Besides the fact that grieving is excuse enough, our friends and family who care about us don't require an excuse to be there when we need them. They do, however, want direction. They *want* to know how they can best be of service—all we have to do is ask. And that help can come in many forms, from cheerleaders to pep us up, to laughter-filled hours that reenergize us, to confidants with whom we can verbalize our fears, to a community's worth of helping hands to fill in all the other gaps.

MOTHER, MAY I?
YES, BUT CALL A FRIEND.

Honestly, I probably should have been respecting my emotional tolerance, cleaning my windshield, and asking for help all along, not just when grief pummeled me, but here I am.

Of course, there are also times when expressing our personal grief must take a back seat so we can care for others. This could look like being present for your parent after their spouse passes or caring for your child as they grieve their grandparent, parent, or sibling. Grief rarely strikes just one family member; instead, it threatens to burn down an entire home.

Which leads me to my next difficult revelation: it is not anyone's responsibility to hide death and grief from children. Like any doting parent, I worry about my children. I want them to have friends, to be nurtured and challenged, and to find interests they are passionate about or just genuinely enjoy. I want them to be kind, confident, and curious. I want them to be happy.

But there is a tendency among modern-day parents to foster exclusively positive childhood experiences, and as a result, they hide away life's more unsavory truths—specifically the existence of cruelty, suffering, and death—for as long as possible. We want to create these beautifully translucent bubbles around our children where childhood naivety can thrive—where, ideally over long periods of time, the bubble develops a small leak that slowly lets in the world's negativity at a rate at which the child can healthily process it.

Except it doesn't always work that way. Sometimes, the bubble is popped all at once by hardship or loss, and then the question becomes how does the reality of the world affect children who have been stripped of their bubble suddenly and/or prematurely?

As Adelaide's older brother, Jackson naturally fell into a caregiver role with her. Not because we asked him to help take care of her, but because that was one of the ways we interacted with her and showed how much we cared about her. He *wanted* to help care for her *because* he loved her. So, I suppose, it felt natural to Jackson that when his sister died, and I was visibly grieving, he would show how much he loved me by trying to take care of me. Sitting with me, hugging me, asking me how my day was. Simple gestures, sure, but they told me he was always aware, always watching me, ready to show care when it was needed.

This role reversal is difficult to swallow and comes with a heavy helping of parental guilt, but maybe it's not as screwed up as society would have us believe. In a perfect world, Jackson, a child, would not feel like he needs to take care of me, his parent. But our world is not perfect, and I have a hard time believing that my son caring for others and being in tune with the needs of those around him is a bad thing. It is just one of the ways that Jackson has learned how to connect with and express his love for people.

A less desirable side effect of this quality is that he rarely speaks of Adelaide without Miguel or me prompting the conversation. He doesn't want to upset us. I have learned, though, that he isn't suppressing his memories of her. When I've asked him to clean his room, or when he is stalling at bedtime, I have found him looking through the memory box we made together before she died, or the photo album filled with pictures of the two of them together—using tools we helped him create so that he could grieve in his own space and time (see chapter four).

Yes, I have been relieved when I could protect Jackson from some of the more abrasive manifestations of my grief, like my side-of-the-highway break-down on our move back to New Jersey. I don't want him to worry about me more than he already does. But that doesn't mean that he doesn't see me cry when something in a TV show we are watching reminds me of Adelaide, or his father when he tears up at the opening notes of "Proud Corazón" from the movie *Coco*, which the Chicago cast of *Hamilton* sang at Adelaide's celebration of life. We want him to know that we still think about her, that her loss still affects us, and that there's nothing shameful about displaying these emotions. My hope is that Jackson understands and learns, from watching Miguel and me, that emotions don't have to be hidden and that grief is as much a part of life as joy.

At some point not long after Adelaide's passing, Jackson started asking questions about who was going to die and when. He was clearly thinking about death, his own as well as mine and Miguel's, more than the average video-gaming or Nerf-blasting child who considers "dead" a momentary inconvenience or delay of game.

I couldn't dismiss his fears because he was all too aware of the cruelty, suffering, and death that is inevitable in our lives. However, I could try and reassure him that none of us were terminally ill like Adelaide had been. His questions were unsettling at first, but the more I thought about it, the more natural it seemed. Don't we all ruminate a little more intently on our own mortality after losing someone close to us? Where my concern grew was when I noticed Jackson becoming exceedingly cautious around anything that had the potential to harm him: amusement park rides, contact sports, trying almost anything for the first time. Perhaps he would always have been this way, though that was not the kid I imagined him becoming when he was climbing up our stairs on the wrong side of the banister at the age of four. But now he is acutely aware of the fragility of life—and once that anxiety-laced gift is unwrapped, there is no way to put it back in its box.

Up to a certain age, I'm fairly certain I told my mother everything. I remember pulling myself up on top of her dresser and watching her change the sheets on her waterbed (ah, the wonders of the '80s). Knowing she was a temporarily captive audience, I'd word vomit every emotion and detail of my life, or book I was reading, or disagreement with a friend. Jackson has never been this kid, despite me buying books for us to read together and asking him questions about the way certain situations or memories made him feel. We filled out a memory book together every night before bed so that he wouldn't forget his memories of Adelaide. Yet he still actively resisted diving much below his surface-level emotions with me.

I desperately wanted to be his person, his safe space—but that was what I wanted, not what he needed.

So, we enlisted the help of professionals. Jackson has actually been seeing "feelings doctors" of one sort or another since he was six years old. Back then, it was so he would have someone to work through the difficult emotions of having a sick sister whose needs often superseded his own. Then there was the social worker who helped him make sense of his sister's impending death. Now, he has a therapist that he can talk to about his sister's loss, our move during a pandemic, the addition of a new sister to the family, and everything between and beyond. As long as he's talking to someone, and that someone is trained and skilled enough to help him navigate his questions and emotions, then it doesn't have to be me or Miguel that he's talking to. Just as we want people to meet us in our grief where we are, we too must meet others grieving where they are. Miguel and I still make sure he knows we are available to talk and listen—and, sometimes, he'll surprise us.

On the second anniversary of Adelaide's passing, I kept Jackson home from school for a family day—one specifically taken to hold space for our mutual grief. We watched videos of Adelaide, looked at pictures, shared memories, and then went to a farm not far from our New Jersey home to pick sunflowers for no reason other than it was a simple and seasonal activity that got us outside and ate up time in the day.

When Jackson went back to school the following day, he asked his teacher if he could share why he had been absent. His teacher graciously allowed the detour to his lesson plan, and Jackson told the class about Adelaide and answered questions about her epilepsy and disabilities. Then other classmates shared about their own losses. That evening Jackson told me it had felt good to share, to be listened to and better understood. To hear from his classmates that they had experienced loss too. (Which goes to show that there are no age parameters on wanting to feel normal in our brokenness.) "Heartwarming" was the specific word he used.

I am incredibly grateful to Jackson's teacher for not only recognizing the moment and allowing a change in class plans, but also for creating an environment where the children felt comfortable sharing. Jackson's bubble burst long before we would have liked it to, and, for better or worse, he may forever live a more cautious life and be more in tune with the moods of others as a result. But as long as he knows he has safe places where he can share, express, and process his emotions, be it at home, a therapist's office, or school, he is going to be as alright as any of us will be following loss.

Worrying about other people in our life while simultaneously stumbling through our own grief can leave us just as drained and dehydrated as crying into a box of wine. But as long as we create the spaces for our loved ones to talk, as long as we listen, engage, and acknowledge their dreams *and* their fears, as long as we meet them in their grief where they want to be met, our loved ones who are depending on us—they will be alright. And so will we, if we listen to our bodies and our hearts and get our permission slips in order.

"Mother, may I?"

"Yes, you may."

What are the symptoms of your emotional hangovers? What (or who) is the leading culprit? What permissions could you request from yourself to limit their impact?

If these prompts don't connect with you, feel free to write about anything that does.

13

When You Feel Like a Deranged Dancing Chicken

> Here is what no one told me about grief: you inhabit it like a skin. Everywhere you go, you wear grief under your clothes. Everything you see, you see through it, like a film.
>
> —Margaret Renkl, *Late Migrations*

Grief is not linear. It just isn't. We can process a provocation, feel the itch of its healing scar, only to have it picked open months later when we least expect it at school pickup or on a conference call. We will ping-pong back and forth between feeling like we've processed something one day—like we're ready to move forward—and feeling like we're back in the dark two days later.

Shortly after arriving in New Jersey from Chicago, we discovered that our moving truck would be delayed by two weeks. Then a literal hurricane hit, knocking power out for a week in the middle of an August heat wave. And as the pandemic raged on, we learned Jackson would start at his new school, where he had zero friends, on Zoom. Every time one trial passed, a new one replaced it, and unfortunately, any progress I'd been making with my grief took multiple steps back with each trial. I was frustrated and overwhelmed at my lack of progress—until a friend who has a chronic illness reminded me I was already a professional at this dance. It had just been that before, it had been Adelaide leading the way.

With each failed med, each hospital admission, each test with inconclusive results, we took a few steps back and then once again set our sights forward. Two steps back, one step forward, two steps forward, three steps back. By framing my grief as a similar dance, just with me leading, fighting for my *own* future, I've been able to wrap my head around this process. Though I must admit, Adelaide's dance seemed much stronger and more graceful than my own clumsy, half-hearted, deranged-chicken-like interpretation.

Grief, stripped down to its essence, is waffling and uncertainty and confusion. It is like playing pin the tail on the donkey, but you're spun around and blindfolded while underwater. You don't know which way is up, let alone where the donkey's ass is. So yeah, sometimes you'll look like a deranged dancing chicken trying to remember which step moves you forward.

And just as I had concluded that I would never take another step forward ever again, our moving truck finally arrived. I inhaled, ready to exhale a sigh of relief that the moving portion of this life milestone was nearing the finish line—but the exhale wasn't the release I had hoped it would be. As the movers brought furniture and boxes inside, I stood near the front door making sure each item was delivered to its correct place. Thriving on organization and craving control, I had placed a sign on each door that matched how I had labeled each box so there were only certain items that needed more direction.

"That bookshelf goes to Jackson's room."

"That rug goes to the basement."

"The IV pole goes to Adelaide's room . . ."

Every time something of Adelaide's came in the door, I held my breath, hoping that the oxygen would release the tightening in my chest. Her things were here, but there was no little girl to own them. Did the movers wonder where Adelaide was? Had they put it together that she was gone? It didn't matter, of course, what they knew or thought—that was my anxiety taking control of my brain. I stood there making jokes with the movers while I wondered if this was what a mild heart attack felt like. My hands were shaking at my sides. Several times, it was all too much, and I went upstairs for an emotional and mental break. A little medication, some water, and a few deep breaths, and I was back at my post. Finally, our stuff was all in, the movers departed, and we were left to navigate the great unpacking. Yet, I still found myself asking myself, *Are we there yet?*

I had hoped that having our belongings in our house would be the miracle salve to soothe my emotional wounds. And it did help some: unpacking kept me busy, I no longer worried about whether our belongings would ever arrive, and goodness knows I enjoy a good organizational task. The biting edge of anxiety had dulled, but even as our home was unpacked, that nagging desire for a destination persisted.

Physically, emotionally, and logistically—basically in every way possible—I knew 2020 was going to be a transitional year, a year of waiting for our family. COVID merely heightened it all a touch (and by a touch, I mean it was as if 2020 took the gnarliest steroids imaginable). Still, I guess I just thought that "there" was finally moving to New Jersey and beginning this next chapter. But even now that we were in New Jersey *and* reunited with our belongings, I was still wondering if we were there yet.

Sure, people say that "life is a journey, not a destination," but wouldn't it be nice if there were like, I don't know, confetti, balloons, and more parties along the way to mark that we were getting *somewhere?* Inherently, we crave a finish line. It is this desire to progress toward some ultimate goal that inspires the choreography for our chicken dances. But the joke is on us—there is no ultimate goal, no final finish line (outside of, perhaps, death) but instead many, many small pit stops along the way. So, we find ourselves subject to life's choreography: endlessly meandering with awkward and jerky motions, forever wondering if we've arrived. We must get better at this dance at some point, though, right?

I remember being told shortly after Adelaide passed that a deep loss never truly leaves you—you just get better at carrying the grief, at learning to live with it. I heard the words, but they didn't compute—how in the world do you just live with this kind of unbearable grief . . . forever? Then I remembered the early days of Adelaide's illness, when we learned she would not have a typical life. We grieved our little girl, her life, and the lives that we had envisioned together. The grief never wholly went away and would resurface with each regression or hospital admission. But I found a way to accept the grief. To live with it. It took years, though, and I still had Adelaide to care for and love on.

Since Adelaide passed, I'd been playing tug of war with this grief, succumbing to it, then trying to reject it, but never allowing myself to accept it. If it took years to accept my grief over the loss of our idealized life *with* Adelaide, then I had to imagine accepting a life *without* her would take even longer.

Here's the thing: grief journeys can be really fucking dark. Pardon my language. Actually, never mind. Don't pardon it; these are powerful feelings and I need powerful expletives to express them. Grief is not a road lined with adorable fluffy puppies and white picket fences. It is dark. Fucking dark.

But there are occasional flowers, and spots of sunshine. And as I grow—as my acceptance grows—I have to believe that the rocky, nearly impossible terrain will slowly get more manageable. *This* is living with grief. It is accepting its permanent presence in my life. Accepting the grief doesn't take the pain away, but it can dull the edges enough so I can get out of bed again tomorrow.

Hi! This is Kelly Cervantes.
I have an 11AM appt and am here now.

You may come inside and
go downstairs.

I read the text three times. Go downstairs. But that was where the ultra-sounds took place, and I wasn't getting an ultrasound. Had they remodeled? Were the ultrasounds moved? Did they know something about my body that I didn't?

Visiting the ob-gyn for an annual exam is not exactly a banner day for any childbearing person, but I dread the downstairs of this obstetrician a little extra. After entering the building, I double-checked at the front desk to be sure they had directed me correctly.

"Yep! Through the door behind you, and the stairs are on the right."

I knew where the stairs were; I knew that the walls in the stairwell were painted pink; and I knew that seven years ago, just two years after giving birth to Jackson, I had lain on a table, my twenty-week-pregnant belly slimed with goo, trying to interpret the sudden silence from the typically chatty ultrasound tech. In the days and appointments that followed, Miguel and I learned that our son Elvis, with whom I was sharing my body, would not survive birth. He had been diagnosed with a rare fatal fetal anomaly, and we would choose to terminate the pregnancy to prevent his inevitable suffering and protect my mental health. At the time I thought this was my life's defining loss and now I should be free and clear of additional major life trauma. I mean, what are the odds that completely unrelated, life-shattering lightning strikes occur multiple times to the same person over the course of a few years?

Don't answer that.

Anyway, I hadn't been to the downstairs part of the office since then, elect-ing instead to have all further ultrasounds for Elvis, and eventually Adelaide, done at the hospital.

| You may come inside and go downstairs.

Holding tight to the railing, I noticed the walls were still pink, but that, yes, renovations had indeed changed the space around to allow for additional exam rooms. My relief was short-lived, though, as I spotted the ultrasound room. The same one, dimly lit so technicians and patients could better view the screens, with photos of the ultrasound tech's healthy children adorning her desk.

"Kelly? You can take a seat in room nine."

I followed the nurse to the exam room, relieved to put a door between me and the ultrasound equipment.

Once the exam concluded, as I was walking out of the building, I congratulated myself for facing multiple anxieties in less than an hour. Go me! Naturally, this called for a well-deserved treat.

I was pulling into the Dunkin' Donuts parking lot before I realized I had left my phone in the exam room. Fuuu . . . You'll be happy to know I survived a return trip to retrieve it.

Back at home, I tried to focus on folding the overflowing pile of laundry while watching a documentary that required little direct attention in an attempt to stop a flood of intrusive thoughts about pink walls. I still had one more social activity that day, a birthday dinner for a friend's daughter at a hibachi restaurant, and I needed to, at a minimum, put on the facade of emotional health.

It took pulling into the parking lot for me to recognize the restaurant. The last time I had been there was when Miguel and I came for our seventh wedding anniversary. That time we had chosen it for the sushi, not the onion volcanos. It also happened to be right after Miguel had booked *Hamilton,* and I was grappling with all the sudden and drastic changes in our life. I remember little about our meal, but on the way out we stopped at a fountain in the entryway and made a wish: that Adelaide would recover from her hypotonia and epilepsy and go on to live a healthy, neurotypical life.

Two weeks later, she would be diagnosed with infantile spasms and, well, you know the rest. So, basically what I'm saying is, don't be rushing off to the wish fountain in the lobby of the Japanese restaurant off Route 22 in New Jersey. The food may be yummy, but their wish-granting fountain is busted.

"Have you been here before?" our friends asked.

"Nope, first time!" Today, lying was easier.

I spent a lot of time reflecting on these two random, same-day encounters. I mean, WTF? If they are signs from Elvis and Adelaide, then I kindly request that they send future ones in a slightly less traumatic fashion. Or maybe they know how stubborn I am, and this was how they thought it'd be easiest to get my attention. In that case, I hear you loud and clear, little buddies!

Divine message or unrelated coincidence aside, what matters is that, despite my anxiety, I survived both events. And even though I went straight to bed after dinner, I was able to not only get out of bed the next morning, but even have a productive day.

A year earlier, the mere *thought* of one of these happening would have sidelined me for the rest of the day. But that day, I had survived them both and was pretty proud of myself. I probably didn't make for the liveliest or most engaging dinner companion, but I'd say overall we can notch that as a win in the Big Step Forward column—especially since the week before had been Adelaide's death day and birthday. (In the inspired words of Gilda Radner's Roseanne Roseannadanna, "It's always something. If it's not one thing, it's another." Or, apparently, some weeks or days, it's all the things.)

These things still suck and sometimes make me feel like my grief has choreographed a shuffle backward—but not letting them control my life is an empowering grand jeté forward. Do I wish to forever avoid that downstairs ultrasound room and highway hibachi wishing fountain moving forward? Abso-freaking-lutely. But should I stumble upon them again, or somewhere or something in their same veins, I know I'll be okay.

When the wounds reopen, as they inevitably will, all you can hope is that you remember the right steps to stitch them up and dance forward. The trick here is to accept that there *will* be steps taken backward. Sometimes they are preventable, but many times they are not, so try not to beat yourself up when they happen. Recognize that it's all part of this awkward choreography. Let yourself dance in place for a while, and when your feet feel solid beneath you, try taking another step forward.

That is the beauty of finding acceptance in the dance, of not letting grief control our lives, and of how, in doing so, we can create our own finish lines. We don't celebrate cross-country moves or surviving trauma-provoking days the same way we do a graduation—but maybe we should. Acknowledge and celebrate your achievements, specifically those that don't come with a certificate.

Then, maybe you won't feel the need to keep asking if you're "there" yet. Right now, you are right where you're supposed to be.

In time, we do get stronger and even more graceful at allowing ourselves space to move backward and forward through our grief. I'm not sure we ever reach prima ballerina status, but I promise you, there is hope for all of us deranged-chicken dancers.

In my recurring nightmare where I'm thrown onstage in a production of *Hamilton* to cover one of the Schuyler sisters, my dancing is catastrophic. It's not much better in real life—awake, asleep, in reality, or metaphorically, my dance steps are awkward. But what has your grief dance resembled? What are the events that have knocked you back or lifted you forward? What are you better at dancing through now that would have landed you on your butt before? Now take a moment and celebrate that growth.

If these prompts don't connect with you, feel free to write about anything that does.

_____

_____

_____

_____

_____

_____

_____

_____

_____

_____

_____

_____

_____

14

When You're Facing Anniversaries and Other Meaningful Dates

> Heroism is endurance for one moment more.
>
> —My fortune cookie

What you need to know about anniversaries:

1. They suck (but you already knew that).
2. The anticipation of the date is often worse than the day itself.
3. It can help to make plans for the day months in advance so that your support system is in place when you need it.
4. If all else fails, it's only twenty-four hours; just survive one inchstone at a time.

This feels like as good a place as any to tackle anticipatory grief. Waiting for a future date or moment to arrive, knowing that it will inevitably knock us off our feet. A warning alarm goes off inside us, shrieking that something challenging is heading our way. It masquerades as a useful tool but is actually the manifestation of forward-focused anxiety.

Look, along with Earth's continuous progression around the sun come unavoidable anniversaries. There are dates that will forever be seared into our mind: birthdays, wedding days, diagnosis days, death days—but they are just that, days. Really shitty days. Worrying about them in advance won't lessen the awkwardness or pain of the days themselves. They are our markers in time, our befores and afters that identify the unfathomable number of years, months, and seconds lived since our existence as we know it was forever altered.

Let the day be what it is, and let how you treat the day change over time to serve where you are at in your journey. Create new traditions or put your head down and plow through the day. Whatever you decide makes the most sense for you this year, this month, this second, do it. But whatever you decide to do, be sure to grant yourself an extra helping of grace. You'll need it.

Seriously, these days suck. Try focusing on what brings you comfort. Create a list of items, songs, books, or activities that you can turn to when these days are upon you.

If this prompt doesn't connect with you, feel free to write about anything that does.

15

When Life Feels Out of Focus

What if grief is a skill, in the same way that love is a skill,
something that must be learned and cultivated and
taught? What if grief is the natural order of things, a
way of loving life anyway? Grief and the love of life are
twins, natural human skills that can be learned . . . In a
time like ours, grieving is a subversive act.

—Stephen Jenkinson

Five years goes by so quickly, yet seems so far away from where we currently stand. Five years was more than all of Adelaide's life. Yet also, within a five-year span, Miguel booked *Hamilton*, Adelaide was diagnosed with epilepsy, I quit my career, we moved from New Jersey to Chicago, we experienced amazing once-in-a-lifetime events thanks to *Hamilton*, I fought harder than I ever thought I could for Adelaide's life until she died in my arms, Miguel transferred to Broadway, a global pandemic hit, and we moved back to New Jersey. I mean, if you had told me all of that would happen before it did, I might have locked myself in a cramped closet, à la *Schitt's Creek's* Moira Rose, and never come out. It's no wonder I recently found a note in my Notes app that read "fuck five-year plans."

Two lifetimes ago, I remember sitting across from my boss discussing plans for my career trajectory. At the time I worked in event planning, so a discussion like this should have been in my wheelhouse—I loved planning, coordinating, and negotiating. But it wasn't. I was a new mom and challenged, in a good way, with work, and that was about all I could handle. In the moment all I knew was that my next stop needed to be an afternoon iced coffee. I never came up with that career plan. (I did, however, get the iced coffee because, you know, priorities.)

Years later, after I'd exchanged career goals for a PhD in Adelaide, her doctors would often ask me about her baseline: meaning what her health, behavior, and ability were like on a typical day. Unfortunately, her health and abilities were so erratic that it was difficult to establish any formal baseline. In time, questions about her baseline made me laugh, but it took me a long time to accept that we had no idea what each day would bring and that there was no reasonable option other than to humbly roll with it. All immediate plans were tentative—as long as Adelaide was doing okay, we would try to be there. Something further out? Can I let you know closer to the date?

So, a vision board for what I wanted my life to look like five years from now? Ha! That's cute.

Our family still fought for improvements, but we also accepted the challenges of the day. Plans were made, changed, and circled back to like a football play designed by the Tasmanian Devil. I learned to let go of what I couldn't control and focus on what I could. We couldn't control her seizures, but we could make sure she was seen by the best doctors. I couldn't always take her pain away, but I could love and snuggle her so she knew she was never alone. I couldn't control her multiple rare diseases, but you better believe I had complete control of her resulting schedule, diet, and medications.

After Adelaide died, I'd exclusively thought of the first half of this lesson: the letting go. Everything felt out of my control, so I abandoned it all, and as a result, my present and future life fell further and further out of focus. I needed to re-center and find things that were within my control, but the pandemic was not helping matters; it is unbelievably difficult to get your bearings when life feels bound to a Tilt-A-Whirl. I felt a lack of motivation to imagine or plan for a future when I was so acutely aware of how little control there was to be had. Why bother?

So, I made my world as small as possible, just what was inside the four walls of our home—which conveniently was all we could see, given the pandemic. I chose a new paint color for said walls, I wrote *a lot*, I helped Jackson with his virtual school. In grief, I lived life hand-to-mouth.

As far as I can tell, our lives are little asteroid magnets, and at any given moment, with little to no warning, a galactic rock can fall into our atmosphere and leave a shattering crater in its wake. We can't predict what will be destroyed—but the asteroids will come, and they will change the landscape of our lives forever.

During Adelaide's life, my world endured a barrage of asteroids. Future thought was impossible because I was constantly trying to survive each impact, knowing another was close behind. After she died, there were fewer asteroids and significantly more time between them, but that didn't make planning any easier. How was I to imagine or dream about a future life in which my child didn't exist? It wasn't denial as much as it was stubborn resistance to a future without her—and at the end of the day, it doesn't take much effort to stop envisioning the future when you are desperately clinging to the past.

This isn't sustainable, though; at some point we do have to think about the future again. Life already asks this of us routinely: what are your retirement plans, new year's resolutions, or holiday celebrations? Though it's taken me years, finally the thought of planning for the future no longer makes me itchy all over. Sure, my heart races and my anxiety kicks in and my guilt-inducing dark side chimes in from the banished recesses of my mind: "Who do you think you are, trying to make plans? Or have dreams? You know how little control you have! You know how everything can change with a text, call, or asteroid!"

But the difference between my planning for the future five years ago and now is that I know the asteroids are out there. I thought I knew they existed before, but I was under the impression that they were rare and fairly rationed. (My naivety was breathtaking.)

So, the asteroids are there, and they can hit at any time and make our world utterly unrecognizable. I don't have my own personal Bruce Willis to blast the asteroids, *Armageddon*-style, out of the sky, but that doesn't mean the future is not worth planning for or dreaming about—that it's not worth making decisions around. It just means we have to be okay with charting a new course if our old one becomes a crater.

As Adelaide's mother, I made life-and-death decisions daily, often with only seconds to weigh my options. Other times, I may have had days to weigh the risk versus reward of a new medication or procedure, but the consequences were no less critical. Whether it took moments or months to assess the returns, I knew I was making the best decisions with the information available to me in those moments. That doesn't mean that I didn't beat myself up when the results didn't turn out as we had hoped. But there also wasn't much time to dwell on disappointment when there was always another crisis, another flash point, waiting around the corner.

When I was truly in my stride as Adelaide's mom, I felt like a master decision-maker for all things in life. The weight of the decisions I had to make for Adelaide's care were so heavy that all other decisions felt, if not trivial, at least manageable. I developed a clarity in perspective around what kind of car to buy, which extracurricular activities Jackson would be enrolled in, what to have for dinner. Decisions that I might have labored over before Adelaide no longer carried the same burden. Of course, they were still important and deserved proper consideration, but they paled in comparison. (Okay, so technically, I've never cared about what kind of car we have, but you get the point.)

By no means do I *ever* wish to have to make daily life-and-death decisions again. Under any other circumstance, i.e., were it not my child's life at stake, the pressure would have been unbearable. But there was no one else better informed to make those decisions, so I had to figure out a way to bear the unbearable for Adelaide.

However, I *do* want to hold on to that perspective and confidence that I had when I was Adelaide's Chief Decision-Maker. Just like I knew Adelaide best, I also know myself and my family best. I can consult with others, as I did with Adelaide's providers, but in the end, I have to trust that I will make the best choice with the information available in the moment. Just like I used to.

So, I created a system to remind me how I made decisions at my peak:

Assess the information,
Make a decision,
Be confident with the decision,
Move on.

Assess, make, be, move.

Broken down, it seems so uncomplicated. **Assess**: What information is available to me and needs to be considered? **Make**: From there, make a decision. **Be**: Now, this may seem like where the process should end, but when carrying grief on your back, decisions rarely rest easy. The second-, third-, and fourth-guessing begins. Doubt settles in, makes itself a drink, and puts its feet up, which is why we must learn to be confident in the decision that we've made. **Move**: Perhaps the most important step is simply to move on. The decision has been made, so now we're on to the next.

My daily decisions are not as intense as they once were, and even though I have more time to dwell, my decision-making superpower is still there. I just need to flex it.

Assess, make, be, move.
Assess, make, be, move.
Assess, make, be, move.

No one wants to be Uncle Rico, stuck in the past reliving his old varsity-athlete glory days. However, sometimes the pull of the past can feel too strong to fight, like a growing mist that blocks out the sharply real present playing out in front of us. A mist that pulls us toward The Hads.

When you are lost in The Hads, what is directly in front of you is blurred as your focus is pulled to what is impossibly out of reach. You *had* a child, a spouse, a mother, a friend. You *had* them in your physical life, and now you don't, yet everywhere you look all you see is their absence. In The Hads, remorse for the should haves, resentment for the would haves and could haves, and remembrance of the what was becomes one indistinguishable and crippling emotion.

The pain can be paralyzing, and as a result it can feel easier—sometimes even vital—to shove it down.

It's one of those days where suppressing feels like the only logical choice. And it's hot—like sitting still and I'm still sweating hot. The pool water reflects the sky, which is the exact color of blue as the crayon named after it. Children laugh and splash, bug-eyed with ill-fitting goggles. A little girl in a bright pink Minnie Mouse swimsuit splashes in the shallow water in front of me. She looks to be about five years old, the same age Adelaide would have been—if she were alive.

I *had* a daughter.

It is summer 2021, the pandemic is limping through year two, and Miguel has yet to return to work as the theaters remain dark. I am months away from meaningfully entertaining the idea of adding to our family via adoption, and we are over a year away from welcoming Anessa. With my parents now vaccinated, we decide it's safe enough to take a road trip and visit them in North Carolina. It will be good to see them, but also, after over a year into quarantine, we are in desperate need of a distraction and change of scenery.

I should be able to relax here, relinquishing some control to my mother while vacationing away from the responsibilities of our typical home life. Except I can't, because everywhere I look I see my daughter. Her absence is as palpable as her physical presence ever was. I see her in memories attached to every room of the house, like my father's office, where she stopped breathing while sleeping on an air mattress on the floor on Christmas Eve. With my mother beside me, watching her vitals on our home monitors, I used an Ambu bag to kick-start her breathing while additional oxygen blew through her nasal cannula from the droning oxygen concentrator behind her. While I squeezed the blue plastic balloon of the Ambu bag, mimicking her breath, I wondered how I would explain to Jackson on Christmas morning that his sister had died the night before.

"Merry Christmas, buddy! Santa came, but your sister died."

Thankfully, that conversation was not realized. Adelaide pulled through the night, as she had so many times before.

Then there was my parent's patio, where I had taken one of my favorite photos of Adelaide. It was her second Christmas; she was wearing a ridiculously fancy red dress even though we had no plans to go anywhere. My brother, Cameron, is more appropriately dressed in pajamas, sitting on the couch beside her and propping her up since she could no longer sit on her own due to the devastating effects of the infantile spasms. In the photo, she has the brightest smile on her face, her hair tied up in a tiny sprout on top of her head, and she is squeezing Cameron's finger. Looking at that photo now, all I can see is pure joy. But I know that at the time I took it, I was dwelling on how all the presents I had opened for her were developmentally for an infant, not the toddler she should be becoming. In the moment, I had missed how happy she was. She didn't care that she wasn't able to stand and manipulate a push toy. She was happy being loved.

Today, though, we have escaped my parent's haunted house of memories and have ventured to the pool. If I thought that would offer me a reprieve from Adelaide's echoes, I was wrong. Minnie Mouse Swimsuit continues to splash mere feet from my lounge chair, oblivious to the world beyond her. Meanwhile, I feel disconnected to the world in front of me and can only focus on what is beyond: Adelaide had played in this pool too. I had stuffed her steroid-injected sausage legs into the holes of a baby float. Unable to support her weight above the water, she had tilted backward as if she were lounging at a spa. All that appeared to be missing was cool cucumber slices over her eyes and an herb-infused water in hand. Of course, her positioning was not by choice, and she was never able to hold a cup or swim independently.

Still, she had been here. She should be here now, splashing and playing just like Minnie Mouse Swimsuit. But she's not.

I had a daughter.

Now I didn't.

Just then, Jackson clumsily surfaces with a diving ring in hand, wearing his own bug-eyed goggles. I remind myself that I *have* a son, but The Hads have already closed in around me.

Look, visits to The Hads are inevitable. Significant people in our lives do not disappear without a trace; their memory is *everywhere*. So, of course we are going to get sucked into The Hads every now and again. The trick is to not get lost in there.

And The Hads are not exclusive to grieving a death. Long before Adelaide's status went from have to had, I struggled with her presence, or lack thereof, at everyday events. I was sitting at Jackson's dance recital, waiting for his hip-hop number while watching the three-year-old ballerinas in their bubblegum-pink tutus.

"Point, touch, plié." The instructor guided the girls through the routine from the floor in front of the stage, their wide eyes glued to her for her next exaggerated movement. Tears poured uncontrollably from my eyes as my two-year-old daughter sat sleeping in the stroller next to me, her emergency medical bag hanging off the handle.

"We do have a child performing in this recital," Miguel reminded me, taking my hand in his.

"I know," I said, pulling my hand away to wipe at my tears. Merely a few sparkling-leotard-filled numbers later, a child of mine would be on that same stage, so why was I focusing on the one who wasn't? Why couldn't I compartmentalize this grief and enjoy the moment in front of me? At that time, Adelaide was still very much a have—but I was already grieving the idealized life I had imagined for her.

What we have can never replace what we have lost. Just because I have a son doesn't mean I stop grieving my daughter. Just because you have a living father or a mother-in-law doesn't lessen the grief experienced from losing your mother.

But the first step to clearing the fog of The Hads is to recognize that you're there. There is no way you are going to find your way out of a place if you don't know where you are to begin with. Again, it's okay to visit The Hads—we all do it! We don't need to feel guilty or ashamed, but we do need to acknowledge that that's where we are and that eventually, we will need to find our way out. Once I put a name to this experience, it became much easier to identify when I had arrived.

It did not, however, help me escape. That has taken time and intentional practice.

First, I must get over the guilt of unintentionally landing there yet again. Then, hopefully, I can isolate the cause of this trip, and acknowledge that whatever it is, it sucks. It sucks that Adelaide can't swim in the pool. It sucks that my best friend from high school can no longer call her mother or that my friend will raise his daughter without his wife. It sucks that your parent won't be able to walk you down the aisle, or that you can't send your friend the meme you *know* they would have loved. It is totally not fair that your brother will never meet your child or that you can never share your grandma's cookies with friends again. It is unbelievably unfair to have to live life without the people we loved the most. To be forced to create new memories without them. Memories that *should* include them, because they *were* here. Once upon a time, we *had* them in our lives.

Let yourself feel those emotions. Cry behind some oversized sunglasses, like I did while staring creepily at Minnie Mouse Swimsuit. By not denying the unfairness of the world, by not forcing those emotions down and denying their authentic and sobering existence, by taking a few minutes to feel them, you can then take some deep breaths and return to the present. We will always see the vacancy left by our loss, but we can also make a conscious choice not to miss out on the life playing out in front of us.

Yes, I had a daughter, I tell myself. But I also have a son.

Not "at least" I have a son. I *do* have a son, and he is living, breathing, and enjoying life right in front of me. What pulls me out of The Hads is that I don't want to look back on this time and realize I missed it because I was so focused on the person I can never have again.

So, you watch the father-daughter dance at a friend's wedding remembering that, not so long ago, you had a father too. Your father may not be able to dance with you, but nothing can take that relationship away from you. Even though the person is physically gone, the relationship lives on. If you lose both your parents, you don't cease to be a daughter. If your only child dies, you don't stop being a mother.

Once this revelation settled into my subconscious, I found that instead of thinking to myself that I *had* an Adelaideybug, I could remind myself instead that I will always be Adelaide's mother. Both are accurate, but while one fills me with desperation and sadness, the other fills me with blinding love and warmth. It doesn't entirely quell the longing I feel while watching the little girl play at the edge of the pool, but it helps me pull my focus back to the fore-ground a little quicker.

The Hads will always be there, lurking in the wings of a dance recital or graduation. Sometimes you will see them coming, and other times they will catch you totally off guard. But no matter what you've lost, The Hads can never claim what you have: an eternal relationship and a present life that is worth noticing and living.

In order to bring life back into focus—whether lost in The Hads, wary of the future, or stuck somewhere between the two—we must ground ourselves in the present, choose a direction, make decisions, and have a goal to work toward. Our dreams and aspirations can be the precise lifeline that we use to pull our-selves out of the dark grief hole into which we've burrowed. What we must remember, though, is that it doesn't mean we've failed if those dreams don't become reality. Or if an asteroid blasts through the atmosphere and knocks them to pieces. Or if we're inclined to change our minds. Go ahead and make plans for life's next inchstones, but be prepared to change course if necessary. At the risk of sounding like a state lotto commercial, a dream can't come true if you don't come up with it in the first place.

Take it slowly, though, because let me tell you, going from a viselike grip on the past to envisioning goals and dreams is a lot to ask of someone. What even are my dreams? What dreams can I feasibly work toward?

You have to start somewhere.

Okay, I know I want a happy and healthy family that honors Adelaide's life. I want to financially contribute to my family again in a meaningful way and have a bright and colorful home with massive closets, ooh and a pool! (Watch out, I'm on a roll now . . .)

If there is one thing the last five years have taught me, it is that I have no idea what the next five years will bring—but that doesn't mean those years aren't worth looking forward to. They will have ups and downs and cratering asteroids and breathtaking sunrises. They will ebb and flow because that is how life goes. (Though I would happily take more flow than ebb right about now.) What matters is that we allow ourselves the space to think about a future—a future where we are content and maybe even happy.

What dreams and goals have you abandoned as a result of your grief? Would you consider going after them again, or have they changed? What are they now?

Remember that these dreams can change with time and lived experience. Keep it simple or go big—you don't have to worry right now about how you achieve them; at this stage, the important part is giving yourself permission to come up with them at all.

If these prompts don't connect with you, feel free to write about anything that does.

16

When You're Ready to Face the Death and Whatever Comes After

They say "Follow your heart" . . .
. . . But I can't follow you where you're going . . .

—Ranata Suzuki

I have tried to write this chapter as gently as possible, but there is no denying the trauma it may stir up. If you're not ready to sit in these moments, that is completely understandable. Come back to it when you are.

Whether sudden or anticipated, death happens. The moment it occurs, or the moment we learn it has occurred, can haunt us for the rest of our lives. There is life before, and life after. You will never forget seeing their body, watching them take their last breath, or receiving that call. People have made notable efforts to forget with drugs and alcohol, but those seconds are seared into our brain forever.

Which might be why I used to bristle when people said to me, "I can't imagine what you're going through," because I knew it wasn't true. Every parent has seen, in their anxiety-induced third-parent-eye, their child getting hit by a car when they are playing too close to the street, or we've seen the caller ID flash with a name that shouldn't be contacting us at this moment and immediately mentally doomscrolled through a hundred horrible reasons for their call. We can imagine it; we just don't want to.

I complained about this sentiment to a fellow child-loss mom once. Her response surprised me.

"But can they really imagine? Do they ever really know what it's like until they've been through a loss this profound?"

She had a point.

Someone can imagine the exact moment of loss, receiving the call, or witnessing the horror, but they can't imagine the lasting effect of the moments before and the forever after. In part because we don't talk about it. I get it, death is not the super-stimulating conversation topic you're looking forward to discussing over a bottle of amazing wine or the comical anecdote you can't wait to share with your friends at brunch. Frankly, dying and the literal death itself also just hurt to talk about.

The final weeks of Adelaide's life were exceedingly more difficult to live through than the first few weeks without her—their single saving grace was that I could still hold her and smell her. No one tells you how excruciating the waiting is when you're waiting for someone to die. When you know the inevitable outcome. When you're done looking for cures and instead praying for peace.

"How much longer can she go on like this?" I asked, tucking a wayward strand of curly blonde hair behind her ear. I hadn't seen her eyes in days. Not since they had been made heavy by syringes full of morphine. She was no longer living, not in any recognizable way. She would moan in pain and discomfort, and then more morphine would be administered, lulling her back into a narcotic-laced dreamland.

"I don't think she has much time left," Adelaide's nurse said, pausing her notetaking. "She is actively dying."

This moment plays over and over in my head way more frequently than I would like. I knew my daughter was dying. She was dying because we chose to stop fighting for her life. I had signed the DNR and called in hospice services.

When modern science failed us, we decided to end her suffering the only way left to us.

At the time, I thought there was a chance she could hang on like this for weeks or longer. I knew that wasn't best for anyone involved, but I was stuck between not wanting to let her go and also wanting to escape this emotional hell, this insufferable waiting room in front of death's door, as quickly as possible. Any sense of relief that the end was near was of course accompanied by guilt because who wishes for their child to die? I knew the grief of her loss would be unbearable, but I was desperate for a change from the stressful anticipation of the waiting.

I knew she was dying . . . *Actively dying* was different, though.

Actively dying meant it was imminent.

The following night, under the low light of a floor lamp, cocooned in my arms as I sat on her bed with Miguel and my mother on either side, Adelaide died. Her breathing became irregular, and then it stopped. In the immediate aftermath, my tears were a cleansing relief. The waiting was finally over. But those tears were merely making space for the grief to settle in.

I know this is not the way grief enters everyone's life. That, for some, death comes as a shock. Your loved one is there one moment and gone the next. No long goodbyes or last words, just gone. But regardless of the details, in order to move forward, we must face those final moments, acknowledge them, and accept them. Otherwise, those hours or minutes will haunt us for the rest of our lives.

Perhaps you think that this chapter would have made more sense closer to the beginning of the book, before the chapters on the months and years that followed Adelaide's death—and if grief was logical and linear, that might be true. But grief is not. Also, I'm not sure you would have kept reading if I had thrown "death happens" in your face right at the top. But mostly, it belongs here—toward the end—because the moment of my daughter's death and the week-or-so window on either side was so traumatic that I buried it for years. I wrote my way through understanding so much of my grief, but those final moments have been too much to revisit. Too much emotion, too much guilt, too much pain, too much life in the presence of death. Facing the moment of death, or the moment we learn of the death, takes a certain mastery over—or, at the very least, awareness of—our grief. You don't need to be fluent in your grief, but I've found a certain level of proficiency is required.

It took me the better part of three years before I was able to face that day, to consciously sit in the memory and recall the details. I forced myself to write a bulleted timeline of everything I remembered in a journal. Not for public consumption, just for me. Because no matter how much I never want to recall that night ever again, I also don't want to forget it. They were our last moments on Earth together, and as painful as they are, I still cherish them. I will never presume to know the true meaning of life, but the pain we feel when life is lost must count for something. If life meant nothing, then it wouldn't hurt so bad. That call, that knock on the door, that last heartbeat wouldn't impact us so greatly.

The more I thought about her death, the more I contemplated what happens after death. I was raised Presbyterian and later earned a minor in religious studies in college. God, spirituality, and faith have fascinated me for years. Though I still appreciate the essence of most faiths, I now consider myself more agnostic. Which makes it difficult to contemplate any sort of "life" after death since it's damn near impossible to not attach religious and societal ideology to it. To be crystal clear, I'm not saying that any particular beliefs are right or wrong; I'm saying, for this conversation, let's focus on the material and observable for a moment.

What we're left with is consciousness, which popular thought says resides in the brain. (Though Dr. Bruce Greyson, in his research on near-death experiences, suggests that the brain and consciousness are likely two entirely separate entities that may not be as integrated as previously thought. His book *After* is a fascinating read for anyone interested in a scientific understanding of the possibilities of life after death.[20]) Thanks to Adelaide, I'm all too aware of how little we actually understand about how the brain works. All of this is to say that no one knows for sure what happens to our mind/consciousness/spirit when our bodies die.

It could cease to exist as well, or . . .

What if some part of our loved one is out there? Energy cannot be created from nothing or destroyed, so our life energy must go somewhere. And if that's the case, then what if there is a way to connect with that energy? Shouldn't we at least try?

I wouldn't say I looked for signs from Adelaide, necessarily, but I wasn't closed off to them. I just didn't know what to look for, or how to interpret them if I did indeed stumble across one. If Adelaide were to send me signs, I assumed she would send me ladybugs—an easy sign to associate with her, as we had called her our Adelaideybug and I had always decorated her bedroom with a ladybug theme. I've only seen ladybugs notably a couple times since her passing: one time was in the bathroom at the grief retreat for mothers who had lost children. There must have been fifteen of them all over the walls and ceiling—a true loveliness of ladybugs, and they remained there the entire weekend. *Okay, my little ladybug*, I thought to myself, *I get it—you know I'm stubborn and needed a big sign to know you are here with me. I see you.*

More frequently though, I will feel her presence when a Frank Sinatra song plays. Adelaide's nurse discovered, not long after joining our family, that Adelaide was not a lover of children's music. She would cry out and fidget at even the beginning notes of "Baby Shark," but if you put on some jazz with a little smooth crooning, she relaxed, even opening her eyes for short periods to take in her surroundings. So, Frank Sinatra, in particular, became a regular soundtrack to our daily life.

The first New Year's Eve after she passed, I was distraught over the realization that we were entering a new year without her. A year that she would never physically exist within. Then as the clock struck twelve, the television program we were watching didn't play the traditional "Auld Lang Syne," but instead Frank Sinatra's "New York, New York." Months later, I was walking down the street, remembering the feeling of pushing Adelaide's stroller, when a truck stopped at the light playing "Fly Me to the Moon."

There was also the time that my friend's psychic told her to tell me to look for signs from Adelaide that had to do with money. Which I thought was odd, since Adelaide was three when she died and had no concept of money. However, just the previous week I had been singing a song to our newly adopted daughter, Anessa, that I had regularly sung to Adelaide, and the toy cash register in the room began beeping. The toy was not turned on and had not recently been played with. The screen was blank, and it kept beeping and beeping until I opened the register and closed it again. Several months later, I was walking on a beach alone, talking to Adelaide in my head, when I found a whole, unbroken sand dollar mixed in with the shards of other shells shattered by the surf.

Were any of these actually signs from her? Who knows. I suppose this is where blind trust, or faith, comes in. However, if I believe that I'm connecting with her and it makes me feel better, does it matter whether it's real or not? As far as I can tell, it can't do any harm. Also, if I'm connecting with her now, then oh my goodness, does that bring me immense comfort to know that we will be together again when my body is gone like hers. If no one can tell me otherwise, then why not lean into the signs, and the hope and the solace they bring with them?

So, I am gradually allowing myself to grow more comfortable with the possibility of consciousness sticking around. After all, no one can prove that some sort of life or consciousness after death doesn't exist. Science has yet to explain consciousness, and stories of spiritual connections and near-death experiences are far too prevalent throughout the centuries and across cultures to be entirely ignored. If it can't be disproven, then it might be possible; not definitive, but possible.

It was around this time, when I was in the thick of my postmortem musings, that I met up with a fellow child-loss mama for coffee. It had been years since she lost her son, but that unmistakable pain sitting just behind the eyes was still there, if you knew to look for it. Since her son's passing, she had made it her mission to help other parents and families of child loss. She eats, breathes, and sleeps grief, trauma, and healing. So, you'd think she would have a solid handle on her own—and she does!

However, she admitted to me that two different health professionals had told her she needed to reconnect with her lost son in order to move forward and find grounded happiness. At first, I'll admit I was confused—what did she mean by connection? Here is a woman who *literally* discusses grief at weekend-long retreats, shares her story and helps others share theirs—of course she's connected to her son. But as we continued to talk, I understood that what she meant by "connection" was something more—be it spiritual or emotional—with her child, *not* with her grief, or the cause that took him.

Prior to this revelation, I thought writing my blog and being open about my grief journey would keep me connected to Adelaide. I thought continuing to advocate for our epilepsy and medically complex communities would keep me connected to her—and while it has helped me to keep her memory alive, it's not actually *her* I'm connecting with. We *can* find ways to keep our departed loved ones a part of our present if we want to, but it takes conscious effort to create this connection.

Just as we take time to nurture our relationships with those physically with us, we can also make space and time for those that are not. For some people, that could be prayer or meditation. For others, it could be taking a walk on a trail you explored together, visiting their grave, or listening to their favorite album. Sometimes it is the site of their last moments on Earth, a ground zero for our pain. The cross on the side of the road where a car accident took some-one's life, or a bedroom left untouched for years. This need for connection, and the calming effect that can result, is part of why humans build shrines or memorials—we want the ability to visit our pain in an established location.

However, we can also create these spaces wherever we are. Last year, I began writing in a journal, all letters to Adelaide, things I wish I could tell her, ask her, and talk to her about—from how much I miss her to some of my anxieties about bringing a new child into our family. I don't write to her often, but the nights that I do, I undoubtedly feel closer to her. It is also on those nights that I am more likely to see her in a rare dream. For someone else, maybe this looks like continuously adding pictures and videos that their loved one would have adored or found funny to a file on their phone. A bittersweet photo album of memories to be shared. Adelaide will never receive my letters, nor can someone else send their photos to a lost friend—but in a small way, this simple act of pointed intention allows us to symbolically share and communicate with our loved ones.

Simply put, death and what comes after is complicated. All of you out there who are unsure of what to believe, I see you. There are no facts here, noth-ing that can be tested or proven. The only thing to do is gradually open your heart to the possibility of connection and see where that gets you.

What purposeful actions can you take to maintain a connection with your lost loved one? Try writing them a letter catching them up on everything you wished they had been around to experience with you.

And, if you're ready, try writing about the moment your person passed or the moment you learned it had happened. Don't force it if you're not ready; like I said, it took me years. But there is power in facing some of our darkest memories. Take back control through your own words.

If these prompts don't connect with you, feel free to write about anything that does.

17

When You're Ready to Be Okay

You will lose someone you can't live without, and your
heart will be badly broken, and the bad news is that
you never completely get over the loss of your beloved.
But this is also the good news. They live forever in your
broken heart that doesn't seal back up. And you come
through. It's like having a broken leg that never heals
perfectly—that still hurts when the weather gets cold,
but you learn to dance with the limp.

—Anne Lamott

Recent efforts to destigmatize mental health and depression created the now-popular phrase "It's okay to not be okay." This is a completely valid and important sentiment and one to which I still cling. Then, I came across an Instagram post by psychotherapist Seerut K. Chawla in which she says, "It's okay to be okay." These five words, eleven letters, hit me with the unexpected force of a wild pitch: It's okay to be okay.

They seem obvious, right? Being okay is the low bar for which we strive. So, why was this sentence having such an impact?

As we grew closer to the second anniversary of my daughter's passing, I realized I was actually doing okay. In fact, I had been doing okay for a while. My struggle lay in acknowledging it. It wasn't like I was out in the world living my best life (YOLO!); I still had bad days, even a bad week now and then. But the heavy weight of depression, the exhaustion, and the painful reminders of our once-familiar life were easing—and that was the problem. After experiencing trauma and extreme loss, being okay comes with its own emotional strings.

I felt guilty and embarrassed. My dark side threw rapid-fire questions at me, not waiting for a response:

By being okay, are you dishonoring her?

Are you forgetting her?

Shouldn't you be mourning her forever?

What will people think of you being okay?

Oh my goodness! First I beat myself up over grieving too much and being a social black hole and now I'm grieving too little? Enough! If right now I'm okay more than I'm not, then I want to go with that. After all, no one is using the volume of my tears to determine how much I miss my daughter. This is not a competition, an evaluation, or test—it is life. *My* life.

The truth is, we can hold both phrases in our minds: It's okay to not be okay *and* it's okay to be okay—the two are not mutually exclusive. Okay is not even a destination; it's more like a gas station where you stop to refuel on a profoundly long road trip. And it is up to us to reframe our internal dialogue in a way that benefits the life we are now leading. Our internal word choice is just as important as the words we put out into the world. We are surviving, not survivors. Instead of moving on, we are moving forward.

Still, moving forward comes with its own guilt. Guilt I felt acutely when we decided to adopt after Adelaide died. Were we replacing Adelaide by bringing another child into our family? Rationally, I knew this wasn't the case, but I also knew we wouldn't be adopting if Adelaide hadn't passed away. Just like someone who is widowed wouldn't be dating and falling in love again if their partner or spouse were still alive. These are wildly emotional truths to reconcile—but we don't have to reconcile them to acknowledge their truth. Life continues, time moves forward; we are not replacing anyone, we are purely adding to our lives, to our families. We are filling the broken cracks in our hearts.

Throughout history, people all over the world have managed to find beauty in the broken. In Japanese culture, one way to do this is through kintsugi, the ancient art of repairing broken pottery by filling the cracks with powdered gold, silver, or platinum.[21] Instead of trying to hide the repair, to make the broken vessel "good as new," the addition of the metal adds personality or history to the item. In fact, some people have purposefully broken their ceramics so that they could undergo kintsugi—and consider them more beautiful afterward. There are entire Etsy shops dedicated to this process.

Of course, this concept was not just limited to Japan. Across Europe, broken objects were once restored via a process called staple repair.[22] A small hole would be drilled on either side of the crack, and metal staples would be inserted to rejoin the pieces. Having an item repaired in this way required a skilled craftsman, which meant it was not cheap. Any item that was being repaired must have had significant value to its owner. Today, there are antique collectors who specifically seek out these broken items, the repairs adding to their allure.[23]

This trend even carries through to modern textiles. Take clothing patches, for example, and how they are used to add to the character of a worn-out jacket, shirt, or pair of jeans. Instead of being tossed, these well-loved items are more than mended—they are enhanced and given new life.

As with mending cracked pottery and ripped denim, the goal of healing our broken selves is not to pretend as if our wounds were never there. Our cracks, our scars are now a part of us. Fill them with gold, affix to them a vibrant or cheeky patch, enhance them with a tattoo. There is no need to deny how these breaks have shaped you. Allow them to become a part of your story.

The modern news cycle can also make it harder to feel okay, no matter how carefully I've applied the gold. I may find a few moments where my personal world feels stable, until I'm reminded with another breaking news alert how unsteady the world is around me. I'm often left wondering why I should get to be okay when so many others are not. (As if learning to live after a deep loss isn't challenging enough.) It can be exceptionally difficult to find our way to okay when it feels like the world is burning down around us. Who are we to be okay amidst wars, racism, and climate change? Twenty-four-hour news coverage does not make for a strong positive mindset motivator.

Yes, we can take breaks from the news and social media—but that is not a permanent solution. So, I've learned to separate the types of okay into the macro and micro. I am not okay that there are war crimes and genocides being committed across the world—that is a macro concern. But on a micro level, in my little bubble, life is generally okay. Occasionally, the macro and micro will bleed into each other, but on an average day, I do not have to let the macro horrors of the world impact the microcosm of my daily well-being. Is this a privilege unique to my Western world circumstances? Absolutely. I can acknowledge that and still be micro okay.

Other times we are afraid to be okay because we are waiting for the not okay to sneak back up on us. I felt this acutely after our second daughter had been living with us for several months. We were settling into life; Anessa had started preschool and was growing more comfortable in our family. One mid-spring day, I was pulling out onto a main road after preschool drop-off, the sun was shining, the weather was warming, and I found myself genuinely smiling—as if that was my natural state.

Is this really our life? This broken, pieced together, but well-adjusted life?

Do I get to be happy now? Or at least okay?

Such loaded questions, because the grief from losing Adelaide is always there. But I can miss her and still be okay, right? I mean, in this snapshot of our life, this day, this microcosm, everything is pretty great.

Naturally, like any good and traumatized person, I immediately started wondering when the next stress-inducing, life-altering event was going to occur. We had never gone long before the next asteroid cratered at my feet, so why would this time be any different?

Which is when a friend pointed out to me that forced negativity wasn't any better than forced positivity or forced gratitude. We shouldn't settle for living in the not okay because we want to protect ourselves from future disappointment or because we think we *should* be not okay.

Regardless, I've lived through too much to believe that there is any sort of equilibrium to our lives. I see no cosmic scale that balances the good and the bad. Just because we've endured difficult times, doesn't mean that we are "due" for happy times. That would only imply that, if we acknowledge and enjoy these happy times, then we are due for bad times next. Unsubscribe. I have to believe there is a randomness to life's events, and whatever happens will happen. Which means there is no point in allowing tomorrow's mystery crisis to prevent us from enjoying whatever is occurring today.

Being okay also doesn't have to be this massive ideological shift. It doesn't mean that you are suddenly going to live life differently or live every day like it's your last because, wow, that is an insane amount of pressure to live up to on a random Tuesday. Especially when we are juggling caring for our family, doctors' appointments, field trips, athletic practices, music lessons, emails, Zoom calls, and getting dinner on the table. I'm over here trying to make sure that we have milk for cereal and coffee in the morning—crossing things off my bucket list just isn't a priority at the moment.

But should it be?

Several months before I lost a dear friend to breast cancer, we spoke about the pressure imminent death places on life. Time pressure is a legitimate type of psychological stress, but it is most often thought of in relation to work-life balance and feeling like there aren't enough hours in the day—not the existential crisis that occurs when there isn't enough time in *life*.[24]

My friend and I came to the conversation from different places, but our takeaway was the same: there is an unimaginable weight that settles over you when time becomes finite. Whether that time is your own or someone else's, there is a desperation to make every moment count. Before someone passes, even an hour away from them can feel squandered or selfish. We rarely regret the time we spent with someone who is no longer here. Our memories with them become precious, seen through rose-colored filters. We forget altogether what we passed up to be with them. After someone dies, our appreciation for our own limited time can feel that much more intense. Hindsight favors the tragic.

So, am I subpar at life because I'm not always reaching for those bucket list moments? Because I'm not forcing myself to be okay 100 percent of the time? Basically, am I doing this life thing all wrong?

What I can say with confidence is that I value life and I am doing my best, just as my friend did. She showed up to the best of her ability with a contagious laugh, a genuine smile, and the absolute silliest sense of humor. She was okay sometimes and not okay at other times.

Being okay doesn't mean that we fill each day with epic Instagrammable moments. It means leaving the door open for them, and for the smaller, more intimate moments as well. We are leaving ourselves open to the possibility of happiness. How you greet it when it arrives is up to you (though I'd recommend you read the next chapter), but being okay is accepting that happiness and grief can coexist.

When discussing acceptance of grief with my friend Bud, he explained to me his idea of the house that grief built:

> *It has a draft and creaks in the rain but it can also be warm and quiet in the sun. Here pain and joy exist, not in competition or in spite of each other, but as siblings. Not one greater than the other, not one with the sole purpose to cancel out the other, but hand in hand[,] knowing that both (and everything in between) are what make us whole. In this home we've built . . . acceptance isn't when you pack up and move out[;] it's when you unpack and move in.*[25]

Only when we come to a place of acceptance of our loss, when we unpack and move in, can we also accept that we are going to be okay. And that being okay is, in fact, on its own, okay. Embrace the beauty in your broken bits, unpack the grief, and let yourself be okay because inevitably the not okay will be back. And if some happy sneaks up on you one day while you're driving around with the windows down and a jam on the radio, give it a big old hug and enjoy the ride.

For a moment, imagine you are guilt-free—not in a serial killer kind of way, but in a momentary grief exorcism kind of way. Now that you are free of your guilt, what is stopping you from being okay? Or, are you already okay and just haven't been able to acknowledge it yet? Write about what okay would look like or feel like for you. How is that different from what you are experiencing now?

If these prompts don't connect with you, feel free to write about anything that does.

_____

_____

_____

_____

_____

_____

_____

_____

_____

_____

_____

_____

_____

_____

18

When You're Ready to Be Happy

God gave us memory so that we might have roses in
December.
—J. M. Barrie, *A Window in Thrums*

Do what you can, with what you've got, where you are.
—Squire Bill Widener, quoted by
Theodore Roosevelt, *Theodore Roosevelt:*
An Autobiography

Nearly three years into my grief, I found myself barreling toward another
invisible wall.

This time around, my public and private selves were more in sync; I felt less
like a shell. I had learned how to better carry my grief, or perhaps I had developed endurance. I was doing okay most of the time, and yet I still felt weighed
down. Perhaps even pulled down.

"Have you experienced many moments of bliss since Adelaide died?"

"Well, um . . . I'm not sure. I must have, right? I mean, it's been nearly three years. It's just that I'm having a hard time finding a moment that isn't also tinged by her absence."

Adelaide's presence was once the North Star that guided every decision I made. Her loss had turned into an anchor. I was struggling to find a way to move forward with her memory and still allow myself the joy in life that we all deserve. It's like every experience, every memory after her death had a filter on it. The degree to which the filter shaded the moment varied, but it was always there, dulling the colors and dimming the brightness. It's not that I was faking happiness when I exhibited it, but it wasn't the same—it felt tainted or impure.

Yes, I knew this was not what Adelaide would want. In fact, at times, I thought I sensed her annoyance or frustration with me. I knew this shift in mindset was entirely on me. That I was preventing myself from achieving some sort of peace with her death, and with that peace, a connection to her spirit, or soul, or energy, or whatever it was I felt rolling its eyes at me from the beyond.

Yes, I knew that this emotional state wasn't benefiting her, me, or anyone else. She was gone; I wasn't hurting her feelings by allowing my grief to mute during life's more joyful moments. The only people I was hurting were myself and those around me when I wasn't capable of being fully present or appreciative.

Yes, I knew I deserved to be happy. That I should be able to experience joy without feeling sad that Adelaide wasn't there to share it with me. That I shouldn't feel guilty that this was an experience I was having that she never would. However, none of these rational thoughts allowed me to cut my tether to the anchor of her loss because that would mean cutting my tether to Adelaide, and that was impossible. So, if I couldn't cut the tether, what was I supposed to do? How did I hold space for and accept my grief while still experiencing joy?

In Judaism, there is a phrase that is shared after a loved one passes: "zikhronah livrakha," which translates to "may their memory be a blessing." I had always loved this sentiment but failed to understand that it was the precise thing I was struggling to achieve. Instead of Adelaide's memory being an anchor, I needed to find a way for it to be my blessing or, because I love a good thematic metaphor, my buoy. I wanted her memory to lift me up, to keep me afloat, to brighten and enhance my life—to be a source of my joy.

Identifying the issue is one thing; figuring out how to solve it, how to turn an anchor into a buoy, well that's another thing entirely. Then, in a conversation with my brother-in-law, I had an aha moment. We were talking about mindset and how we can grow so comfortable in our own personal chaos or hardships that it can be difficult to break the cycle long after the circumstances that sparked that mindset are over. For him, it was low energy and motivation resulting from a difficult marriage. However, even after the divorce negated his go-to excuse, he still has had to work to break out of that defeated mentality—to make forward progress in his life.

For me, even though I'd actually broken free from depression's chemical effects months ago, the limitations depression placed on my life had become a known quantity to live with and work around. Without those boundaries, the world and all its options felt too vast. Consistent happiness was unknown and scary. So, I sacrificed potential happiness for the comfort of the sadness I knew.

In no way am I saying that anyone can wake up one morning and choose to not be depressed. It doesn't work that way. Thankfully, my depression is situational: I will likely go in and out of it for the rest of my life, but it is not a constant chemical imbalance the way it is for some people. Regardless, I didn't just choose to make the depression go away—it took a lot of work and medication. And even once I was no longer depressed, I still had to make the choice to be happy. To make changes to my lifestyle that reflected depression's lifted veil.

We cling to these self-identities and perpetuate them: the grieving mother, the broken husband. We can't snap our fingers and break out of these cycles, but we can make the choice to take the first (terrifying) step forward. The situations that constrained our life, that hurt us, may not have been our fault, but choosing to be happy is our responsibility.

It was around this time, as I was questioning my alchemical abilities to turn an anchor into a buoy, that Carole's email popped up in my inbox.

Carole Mac is a friend of a friend who wrote the children's book *The Gift of the Ladybug* about accepting her son's illness and his short life. Her creative ventures have not ended there, though. She was at the time producing the pilot episode of *Food Bliss*, a TV show where, as the host, she planned to give guests a culinary experience that dreams are made of to help them find and feel joy again after deep loss. Think Anthony Bourdain meets *Queer Eye* (minus the physical makeover and five gay stylists): travel to a part of the world and experience their delicious food in hopes of finding moments of bliss—an act that is exceedingly difficult to do once grief has descended upon your life.

"I want you to be my first guest—to come with me to Sicily to film the pilot. Is that something you would be interested in? Something you could do? Can I try to help you find moments of joy again?"

"Um . . . yes?"

It sounds like a no-brainer, right? I mean who says no to an all-expense-paid trip to Sicily with the sole purpose of finding happiness in wine and food? Not me! That's for damn sure. Or at least not me once I processed all my guilt around deserving the trip and leaving my family . . .

After touching down in Sicily, we drove an hour up the coast, watching Mount Etna, an active volcano, smoking out one window while the Mediterranean Sea crashed on the rocky shore out the other. At this point in my grief journey, I wasn't crying over Adelaide daily, sometimes not even weekly, but there was no holding back the tears now. It was all just so freaking beautiful. I had never seen anything like it all before—but I was also registering that this trip wouldn't exist without Adelaide's death. How could something so stunning, so dreamy come out of my ultimate tragedy? There was no reconciling the two, so I did my best to simply accept it and stay present.

Still, by the time I stepped into my room, with the summer Italian sun blazing in the window, luggage at my feet, and jet lag from a sixteen-hour journey in my bones, I questioned what in the hell I had gotten myself into. It suddenly dawned on me that I didn't even know these people, and I barely understood what we were doing there. Who had I just surrendered temporary control of my life to, and what exactly was I surrendering for?

Over the next four days, I learned that the answers to these questions were as complex and varied as grief itself.

Surrendering control of my circumstances was the easy part. I gotta say, not being the cruise director for four days and simply showing up when and where I was told was *ah-mazing*. It also helped considerably that the people I had surrendered control to were exceedingly kind, compassionate, and talented.

Having never visited Italy before, I was completely taken aback by the next-level hospitality exhibited by everyone from the butcher who taught me how to make traditional Sicilian sausages, to the shepherds who boiled fresh ricotta before my eyes, to the winery owners and managers who gave me tours of their vineyards and shared their delicious wines. There was the Mamme del Borgo (oh the mamas!) who taught me to make pasta and showered me with love and hugs in a way that only mamas can. There was the baker who demonstrated the ancient way of making granita and made the most delicious cannoli I have ever tasted in my life, and our absolutely delightful bed-and-breakfast hosts, makeup artist, and sound professional, among many, many others.

Amidst the people of Sicily, I found a warmth that went far beyond anything I ever expected from strangers who were teaching a silly American how to create the dishes and wine they make and drink daily. But the moments between the shots were equally soul-filling: wandering around small mountain villages on my own, putting my feet in the Mediterranean Sea, and chatting about all things grief with Carole on drives through narrow mountain roads. Having lost a child herself twelve years before, she showed me that happiness was achievable. That I could still love and honor Adelaide while also having joy in my life—that contrary to prior belief, the two were not mutually exclusive. I mean, when the world around you appears so epically different from anything you've experienced before, it's sort of difficult to not let it transport you mind, body, and soul.

I had done all my mental prework to be sure that I didn't feel guilty about being away. I was truly enjoying the trip and doing my best to stay present when Miguel called on Sunday evening to tell me he took our daughter Anessa to the hospital with a virus and low oxygen. Surrendering to the experience was one thing; surrendering control of my family's health felt obnoxiously ironic. But an ocean away, there was nothing I could do. Given Anessa's otherwise healthy constitution, and Miguel's regular check-ins, we knew this was simply a severe cold in a little girl unable to clear the junk in her lungs. She was going to be okay. I heard that said to me, and said it to myself, and knew it was true in a way it never was with Adelaide.

As much as I wanted to be with Anessa, that was not an option. Even if I could have made it back across the ocean, my presence would not have made a difference in her health—Miguel would have appreciated the reduction to his stress level, but he was not incapable of managing the situation. I also surprised myself by feeling relieved that this was one hospital visit I did not have to manage. Being back in the hospital with a child struggling to breathe would have brought back some serious PTSD. I would have powered through because that is what parents do, but it would have come at a cost to the emotional and mental progress I'd made. In this situation, given our history, Miguel was better suited to managing this one, and I *never* would have accepted that had I been home.

By being honest with myself, even though Anessa was in the hospital, I was able to surrender to the joy—no, the *bliss*—of my Sicily experience. I allowed myself to be in the moment, to enjoy the land, the people, and the food. Of course, there were moments when I questioned what in the hell I was doing not rushing to the airport and demanding to get on the next flight home, but in the end, I always came back to the rational truth that my presence would not have changed the situation.

If I could surrender control, stress, and grief for a few days in Sicily—albeit with stunning and engaging distractions that are so wonderfully far from everyday life—then, perhaps, I could also surrender them when I was home. To be clear, my days in Sicily were finite and a literal world away from my life in New Jersey. Surrendering control of my schedule and the ability to be physically present for my currently ill but otherwise healthy child is not the same as surrendering control and accepting that I couldn't make my other child healthy and that I will never be able to hold her again. The two situations are not the same, and so I will not hold myself to what I will now refer to as my "Sicilian standard" because, inevitably, I will disappoint myself. I can live with the goal of allowing myself to experience unencumbered happiness and also acknowledge that I am human, that grief is not linear, and some days my Sicilian standard may be more difficult to achieve than others. The goal is not to be happy all the time—that is as unhelpful as it is unrealistic. Instead, my goal is to allow myself to feel happiness without a grief anchor weighing me down. The important takeaway from Sicily was that I now knew that I could do it. I could be happy again. I could surrender to joy. I could find my bliss. Regardless of my surroundings, if I could do it once, I could do it again.

Now, I realize that not everyone has the opportunity to fly halfway around the world to enjoy a four-day adventure curated with the direct intent of helping them find moments of bliss. We can't all *Eat, Pray, Love* our way to happiness (though should that be an option, I *highly* recommend it). That said, we *can* carve out time for ourselves where we temporarily remove the responsibilities of everyday life. Ideally, we use that time for an experience that doesn't already have memories of our lost loved one attached. Maybe it's a weekend away with girlfriends or a solo night at a hotel. Maybe it's taking a free class at your local library, picking up a new hobby from YouTube, or exploring a new hiking trail. Anything to break the monotony of everyday life, pull you out of the mundane, and force you to surrender to something new.

Happiness doesn't have to be elusive. In its purest form, it is one of the simplest emotions ever experienced. Here I had been trying to chemically alter an anchor into a buoy when I'd forgotten that every buoy bobbing above the surface of the water is held in place by its very own anchor tethering it to the ocean floor. I didn't need to turn my anchors into buoys; I needed to tie a buoy to my anchors and let go of both. With a buoy acting as a marker, I can revisit my anchors when I want to or need to. They are not lost to me, but they are also no longer weighing me down or holding me back. *Nothing* can sever our love with and for those that have passed; worrying that something could is wasted energy. It is up to us how we deploy that love, and, as far as I can tell, there is no better way to honor love than to live our own lives, for as long as we are fortunate to have them, as fully and happily as possible.

Wanting to feel happiness again and allowing ourselves that experience are two different intentions. What are the anchors preventing you from experiencing happiness? What are the connections and actions you can make and take to tie your grief anchor to a buoy, allowing your loved one's memory to be a blessing?

If these prompts don't connect with you, feel free to write about anything that does.

_____

_____

_____

_____

_____

_____

_____

_____

_____

_____

_____

_____

Epilogue

There is a sacredness in tears. They are not a mark of weakness, but of power. They speak more eloquently than ten thousand tongues. They are the messengers of overwhelming grief, of deep contrition and of unspeakable love.

—Unknown

It's one of those days where my emotions are anxiously pacing just under the skin, tapping me every few minutes to remind me they are there. As I fill my coffee cup. While I prepare the children's lunches. When I return to a quiet house after drop-off. Tap, tap, tap—*all is not well*, they say. I inhale deeply, a futile attempt to drown them in fresh oxygen. By mid-morning, I recognize that tears are inevitable, and holding them back is wasting energy. I can't pinpoint what provoked their onset, but it doesn't matter. It would all come back to her. It always comes back to her.

I taste their salt as they roll over my lips. It's been a while since I've cried like this. The days of crying every day, multiple times a day, of grief exorcisms on the bathroom floor are now as much a memory as my days with Adelaide. The tightness in my throat hurts, but in a good way. I've needed this relief, this release. My surroundings fall away, and it is just me and the pain.

I miss you so much, my Adelaidey, so freaking much. I have found a way to be happy now, something I never thought I would be able to do without you. But it doesn't take the grief away. I want more than ladybug mementos and photograph memories. I want more—I want more; I want you.

And then it passes. The tightness in my throat and the weight on my chest leave me as quickly as they arrived. Tears released seconds ago still travel their paths down my face, pooling under my jaw before falling into my lap. I take a few steadying breaths, allowing the world to fill back in around me. The lawn mower buzzing across the street, a bird cawing in a distant tree. The sun continues to shine; the world continues to spin.

My life did not end with you, even though at times I felt like it should. I will live because I can, because I understand how precious life truly is—even a broken life. Pieced back together with gold paste, metal staples, and bright colorful patches, I will chicken dance on.

Acknowledgments

"Acknowledgments" doesn't quite cover the utter, all-consuming grate-fulness I feel for the people who helped make this book a reality. There is nothing forced about this gratitude.

To Courtney Paganelli and LGR for taking a second chance on me: I wouldn't even be writing an acknowledgment page without your dedication, knowledge, and grounded advice. To editor, meme-sharer, and writing cheer-leader, Alyn Wallace—you have made me a more critical thinker and a better writer. Everyone who has read this far should be thanking you and CE extraor-dinaire, Leah Baxter. To the entire BenBella team for being incredible partners on this publishing journey: I've rarely felt more professionally supported.

To Marcelle Soviero, for your crash course in memoir writing and encour-aging me all along the way. To my early readers: Wendy, Bud, Carole, thank you for bringing your varied experiences to these pages. And especially to Terry, for being a positive guiding force since I was fourteen years old. I am better for knowing each of you, and this book is better for having had your eyes on it. Mary Katherine Backstrom, thank you for being my publishing-world mentor, girls-trip enthusiast, and belly-laugh inducer. To my *Inchstones* readers, your encouragement, compassion, and feedback is the reason I ever had the courage to write this book. To my Hayden's House Mamas, thank you for showing me how normal it is to be broken and that there is beauty and companionship to be found in that normalcy.

A special shout-out to Lin-Manuel Miranda and the cabinet: Tommy, Alex, and Andy for creating *Hamilton: An American Musical*, and entrusting my husband with the title role. The job gave our family the financial freedom to allow me to care full-time for Adelaide during her life, grieve her after her death, and subsequently write this book. To Tommy Kale and Jeffrey Seller for always being in our corner and giving us every kind of support we needed to grieve and heal.

A heartfelt thank you to Eileen LaCario and the team at Broadway in Chicago, as well as Michael Schultz and his Fairgrounds Coffee & Tea company, who helped us put together a perfect celebration of life for Adelaide along with a team of our friends from across the country who coordinated the details.

For years I have leaned on friends for support, time, and favors. Thank you to our friends and family in Chicago, who caught us when we fell and supported us when we tried to stand again. And also, to our friends, new and old, in New Jersey who welcomed us back with open arms and gave us the space to relearn how to walk in our newest normal. There are two friends in particular who took on the heaviest loads. I cannot imagine surviving the early days of Adelaide's diagnosis without my nightly texts with Courtney Rabb. Thank you for being a sounding board and for meeting me emotionally, wherever I was, with honesty and zero judgment. Then there was Jackson's second mother, who stepped up in ways that would never have even crossed my mind. What do you call a person who forces you out of your house when you need it most, but meets you there when leaving is impossible? Who drives you to your psychiatrist appointments, but never treats you with kid gloves? Who loves you and your family unconditionally, but never lets any of you take yourselves too seriously? You call them a Jenny Lane—and you call them often.

To Adelaide's army of nurses, therapists, and medical providers: thank you for caring for Adelaide as if she was your own. Katie—knowing you were caring for Adelaide calmed my mind, but it is your continued support of Jackson that soothes my soul. Nurse A—Adelaide's love and trust for you was not only apparent but unparalleled. Dr. Marcuccilli, Dr. Tobin, and the Rush medical staff, together you added months, if not years, onto Adelaide's life. There is no thank-you grand enough to encompass the gift of time. To CURE Epilepsy and the greater epilepsy community for holding us up and helping us to keep Adelaide's memory alive—thank you for giving me a purpose beyond Adelaide and for being a continued source of hope even on our darkest days.

Thank you to our family: Mary, Mike, Marcos, Martin, Cameron, Danielle, and especially to my parents, Kathy and Doug, for all their love and support (and Cam and Danielle for the legal advice). Mom, thank you for instilling in me the importance of mental health and also for sleeping on a fold-out couch for over a month while taking care of our family during Adelaide's final days. Dad, thank you for passing on your writing genetics, the extensive movie and music exposure, and the hugs—every single hug.

Miguel, thank you for never rushing my grief even when yours was further along. Thank you for filling in the gaps in our home when I was at my worst, even though you weren't far behind me. Thank you for growing forward with me even when our grief wanted to drive us apart. We are surviving together, and there is no one I would rather survive with.

My children are the lights in my life: Jackson, you are my lighthouse in the storm. Anessa, you brought sunshine back into our home. And Adelaide, who is and will forever be my North Star. To my Adelaide: thank you for revealing to me what love means, for teaching me why love matters, and for showing me love's power. You were all at once perfect and broken. My very own kintsugi. I promise to never stop living as long as I'm breathing, and to always look for your signs. I love you, my Adelaideybug, and forever after.

Endnotes

1. Kira M. Newman, "How Journaling Can Help You in Hard Times," The Greater Good Science Center at University of California, Berkeley (August 18, 2020), https://greatergood.berkeley.edu/article/item/how_journaling_can_help_you_in_hard_times#:~:text=The%20people%20who%20journaled%20saw,percent%20were%20comfortable%20doing%20so.
2. Mark Twain, *Which Was the Dream* (University of California Press, 1967).
3. Marilyn A. Mendoza, "When Grief Gets Physical," *Psychology Today* (September 4, 2019).
4. Ibid.
5. Steve, Leder, *The Beauty of What Remains* (Avery, 2021).
6. Kenneth J. Doka and Terry L. Martin, *Men Don't Cry, Women Do: Transcending Gender Stereotypes of Grief*, 1st ed., Series in Death, Dying, and Bereavement (Routledge, 1999).
7. Kenneth J. Doka and Terry L. Martin, *Grieving Beyond Gender: Understanding the Ways Men and Women Mourn*, 2nd ed., Series in Death, Dying, and Bereavement (Routledge, 2010).
8. "Ashley Judd on Mental Illness, Her Mother's Death, and the Importance of Grief Support," July 26, 2022, in *Healing with David Kessler*, podcast.
9. Ellen Hendrickson, "Six Tips for Handling Survivor Guilt," *Psychology Today* (Nov ember 22, 2017).
10. *APA Dictionary of Psychology*, American Psychological Association.
11. Elisabeth Kübler-Ross, "Kübler-Ross Change Curve," EKRFoundation.org, https://www.ekrfoundation.org/5-stages-of-grief/change-curve/.

12. Kate Wong, "Why Is *Homo sapiens* the Sole Surviving Member of the Human Family?" *Scientific American* (September 1, 2018), https://www.scientificamerican.com/article/why-is-homo-sapiens-the-sole-surviving-member-of-the-human-family/.

13. Ayako, Wada-Katsumata, Jules Silverman, and Coby Schal, "Changes in Taste Neurons Support the Emergence of an Adaptive Behavior in Cockroaches," *Science* (May 23, 2013).

14. J. Moll, F. Krueger, R. Zahn, M. Pardini, R. de Oliveira-Souza, and J. Grafman, "Human Fronto-mesolimbic Networks Guide Decisions About Charitable Donation." Proceedings of the National Academy of Sciences 103, no. 42 (2006): 15623–15628, doi:10.1073/pnas.0604475103.

15. Tara Parker-Pope, "Writing Your Way to Happiness," *New York Times*, January 19, 2015.

16. James W. Pennebaker and Joshua M. Smyth, *Opening Up by Writing It Down: How Expressive Writing Improves Health and Eases Emotional Pain*, 3rd ed. (Guilford Press, 2016).

17. Mark Baxter and Paula Croxson, "Facing the Role of the Amygdala in Emotional Information Processing," Proceedings of the National Academy of Sciences 109, no. 52: 21180–21181.

18. C. Daniel Salzman, "Amygdala," *Encyclopedia Britannica* (September 8, 2022).

19. Elisabeth Kübler-Ross, *Death: The Final Stage of Growth* (Scribner, 1997).

20. Bruce Greyson, *After: A Doctor Explores What Near-Death Experiences Reveal About Life and Beyond* (St. Martin's Essentials, 2021).

21. Kelly Richman-Abdou, "Kintsugi: The Centuries-Old Art of Repairing Broken Pottery with Gold," www.MyModernMet.com (accessed May 22, 2022), https://mymodernmet.com/kintsugi-kintsukuroi/.

22. Isabelle Garachon, "From Mender to Restorer: Some Aspects of the History of Ceramic Repair," paper presented at Interim Meeting of ICOM-CC, Corning, NY (2010), https://www.researchgate.net/publication/260158211_'From_mender_to_restorer_some_aspects_of_the_history_of_ceramic_repair'.

23. Andrea Codrington-Lippke, "In Make-Do Objects, Collectors Find Beauty Beyond Repair." *New York Times*, December 15, 2010.

24. Andrew Denoven and Neil Dagnall, "Development and Evaluation of the Chronic Time Pressure Inventory," *Frontiers in Psychology* (December 4, 2019).

25. Bud Hager, "Moving In," *Inchstones* by KC, www.KellyCervantes.com/blog /moving.

About the Author

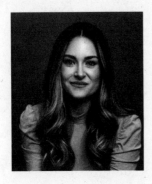

Kelly Cervantes is a writer, speaker, and advocate best known for her blog *Inchstones* and her work with the nonprofit CURE Epilepsy. She has been published in the *Chicago Tribune,* the *Chicago Sun-Times,* and *Cosmopolitan,* as well as quoted in the *New York Times, CNN,* and *People.* Born and raised in the Midwest, Kelly currently resides in Maplewood, New Jersey, with her family and two dogs, Tabasco and Sriracha.